THE ESSENTIAL MOVEMENTS OF T'AI CHI

John Kotsias

The Essential Movements
of T'ai Chi

Library of Congress Cataloging in Publication Data
Kotsias, John, 1948-
The Essential Movements of T'ai Chi

1. T'ai chi chuan. I. Title.
GV505.K64   1984   796.8'155   84-11335
ISBN 0-912111-04-6

Paradigm Publications
44 Linden Street
Brookline, Massachusetts 02146

ISBN 0-912111-04-6

Copyright © 1989 John Kotsias

Table of Contents

Preface

This is a beginners' book, and in T'ai Chi we are all beginners. The theory and exercises in this book can be done by beginners and advanced, young and old, strong and weak.

This book is for everyone who wants to learn T'ai Chi. The most important part is that you do the exercises, do them with principle, and do at least a little every day.

I wish to thank my teachers, my students, family, and friends who patiently encouraged this work.

Introduction

It is noticeable that practitioners of Asian martial arts tend toward conservatism in their training, with marked reluctance toward any new methods, either in techniques or interpretations. This may be the result of habitual references to the legends of the past and the thousand year old classics which are the canons of the arts. These classics, sustained through the centuries, are intrinsic components of a cosmological structure. In time, the arts themselves became a synthesis of the many aspects of the culture. Indeed, the very rhetoric became cryptic and hallowed. All this reflects the setting and context of feudal epochs.

The words and teachings became scripture and many techniques were observed ritual. Rank became important in teaching and the school became monolithic in structure and policy. And thus it came to be that there was scant room for innovations, new departures, or basic polemics. Any new thought can be relegated to negligence or insufficient digestion of the classics.

However, from a scientific perspective, new geography, new economies, new cultures and new inventions can and do add or detract from any traditional system however honored. Progress, expansion, or transformation must proceed in this direction. Hence this book, written by a young Westerner on T'ai Chi Ch'uan and the internal martial arts, is indeed greatly welcomed. The recording of his experiences and his observations in this volume is a definite contribution to the widening understanding of the discipline.

The author, John Kotsias, is a good friend. I know that he is a linguist, professor of mathematics, a passionate martial artist, an exceptional practicing humanist. He combines these attributes with an obsessive desire to widen the spectrum of T'ai Chi Ch'uan without sacrificing the classical virtues. I feel very little urgency to comment on the text itself, as that exercise might obscure the important focus, which is to encourage fresh input toward the universal flowering of the art of T'ai Chi Ch'uan which millions have considered the greatest physical culture system ever devised and which the Chinese regard as the jewel of their integrated culture. I do believe quantitative to qualitative changes occur as more people and minds and cultures participate in this great system of human betterment. Kotsias' book is part of that process.

Marshall Ho'o

Marshall Ho'o

The Old Men
of
T'ai Chi

Professor Huo

Tai Chi is for old men. By age twenty-two I had spent some time studying T'ai Chi, but I devoted most of my time to Karate and Kung Fu. The soft forms of T'ai Chi were for weaklings as far as I was concerned.

Some of my martial art friends had begun studying the Yang family form, a so-called secret style of T'ai Chi Ch'uan with an old Chinese professor named Huo Chi Kwan. No one knew how old he was. His features were smooth and his skin soft, but by the looks of his hands, he was ancient.

I had always wondered how I could learn anything from people over fifty, since most of them have a hard time climbing a flight of stairs. Yet, I had heard some of my teachers speak about the great expertise and power of old masters who progressed as they got older. I didn't believe it!

I went to see Professor Huo Chi Kwan because heavy sparring had begun to take its toll on me. I heard that T'ai Chi had miraculous healing powers, and I felt this would be a good way to cure my injuries and strengthen my weaknesses. I could then return in a healthier condition to competition Karate. So, with all the confidence and wisdom possessed by any twenty-two year old and with a

1

lit cigarette hanging from the side of my mouth, I knocked on the door of Professor Huo Chi Kwan. It was December 12, 1970.

The old man who answered was dressed in his Northern Chinese attire, all white, and in a grey cardigan sweater with six buttons, some buttoned, some not.

"Are you Professor Huo?" I asked as he opened the door.

He muttered a soft reply in a dialect of English that was almost incomprehensible. "Heh, Heh. Just a minute," and before I knew what happened, the door was shut.

About three minutes later, he opened it again. His right hand held an empty glass, and his left hand snatched the cigarette from my mouth, extinguishing it in the glass. It all happened so quickly, yet so slowly. So slowly, that I can still remember the pale color of the single light bulb hanging from the ceiling of his bare, austere apartment in Hyde Park, Chicago.

"I'm a friend of Mr. Foster," I said.

"Oh." His reply came in a very soft voice. "Foster. Mr. Foster. Nice man. Coming soon. Sit down, heh, heh."

I sat in an old wooden chair next to an old wooden table with a green tablecloth covered with many sizes and types of Chinese calligraphy pens, ink tablets, and inks. Some rice paper with some newly written calligraphy was laying across the table top. He rolled it up and sat down at the long end opposite my own.

He looked at me, smiled the most curious smile I'd ever seen, and out of his mouth came those strange utterances again. "Heh, heh." I smiled back.

"I'd like to learn T'ai Chi."

His smile vanished. "Uh?" he said.

"I said I would like to learn T'ai Chi."

The tea pot in the kitchen began to whistle in perfect time so that my question went unanswered. He attended to the tea. He was in the kitchen for four or five minutes and kept walking back and forth, looking very busy.

When he finally came back, I stood up. By then I had realized that he was a very cultured gentleman and I had to use my very best

2

manners if we were to communicate at all. He brought only one cup and the tea had the most delightful aroma I had ever smelled. It was as though I was in a field of jasmine flowers at their peak of bloom. It smelled more like perfume than tea and though I knew it was much too hot to drink, I didn't resist. I knew I had to have a sip.

He was soft and gentle, yet something about his body gave the appearance of being carved from stone. As he returned to his chair, I waited for him to sit down. I took a sip of tea and it seemed that my tension had released from my entire body. Yet somehow I was still in a state of limbo, for it had become obvious that he wasn't going to talk about T'ai Chi. So we talked about the weather and the many paintings that covered his walls.

The entire scene lasted about thirty minutes. I had the appointment at four. Foster was to come too, but he showed up at four-thirty. When he arrived the Professor told him to sit down in a chair that was against a wall near a big bay window that opened up on to a tiny terrace. We put our coats on a bed in the far corner of a living room that measured sixteen feet by fourteen feet. This is where the classes were to be held.

The Professor put the tea on the table for Foster and Amato, but before they could drink it, he told us to change. We did so, each in turn, in a tiny bathroom that was the only other room save for a small walk-in closet. We started our lesson by doing the first three movements of the basic movement of T'ai Chi Ch'uan. The lesson lasted one hour and it contained only these movements and a discussion of basic principles. The next class was to meet the next Monday at four.

After that day, although I knew nothing about this new form of T'ai Chi I was learning, and though I knew very little about the nice old man called the Professor, I never studied another hard martial art, nor practiced any, nor wanted to. T'ai Chi was fun. It had a flavor I could taste in my mouth like no other flavor I had ever tasted. It was wonderful. I didn't care if I could use it to fight, or if the Professor was a good boxer. T'ai Chi was beautiful! It made me feel good. It made me smile.

The next week I went to class a half hour early. I had practiced my T'ai Chi every day without fail, and the idea of learning a new movement was exciting. That week we learned one movement doing it balanced on one leg with non-stop, slow, and exacting repetitions. It hurt, but the hurt felt good. Indeed, it was still a paradox to me that these painful movements, once completed, made my body feel so good.

Eventually my lessons were private, often it felt as though we were in our own little universe. Even the dust on the floor, the plants in the room and the light bulbs took on a entirely different appearance. Practice had become for me an oasis of knowledge that brought light into the rest of my life.

The Dragon of Morse Avenue Park

I studied this way with the Professor for about fourteen months. I changed my mind about T'ai Chi being for old people and I came to believe in the power and strength of old men. Never, though, did I think I would come to believe in dragons as well! Yet, I learned a dragon did indeed live in a park on Morse Avenue in Rogers Park, Chicago. His name was Tsao Li Ming.

One afternoon I went there to visit him. Soon after I arrived, I saw an old Chinese man with a cane and a straw hat approaching. He looked very frail and the hair in his nostrils and his two front teeth gave the appearance of an old dragon that had lost his fire. I wondered how this could possibly be a T'ai Chi Master. This old man looked as if he had trouble standing and I was sure that if the wind came in too briskly off Lake Michigan, he'd be blown across the park.

He went to a bench and sat down. Three strong-looking young men approached him, apparently wanting to learn some martial arts. They gestured in certain ways as if they wanted to "play" T'ai Chi. But the old man put out his left hand, vibrating it side to side, and said in atonal English, "Nohhh. Nohhh."

Not being able to communicate, the three young men left. I still hadn't recognized that this was a T'ai Chi Master, but curiously enough, I approached him and observed him reading a Chinese book with pictures of T'ai Chi postures. I smiled and greeted him and pointed to some of the characters in the book, pronouncing them in my very poor Chinese accent. He looked up, grinned, and with a slightly open mouth said, "Ehhhh."

Standing up, he took off his straw hat and put it down near his cane. He walked into the park, beckoning me to follow. I stood behind

4

him, knowing we were to begin doing the form. As he prepared, this frail old man began to expand and as he expanded he got straighter and straighter and smiled more and more. Everything about him brightened, and then he began to move. To this day I have never seen anyone move as smoothly, softly, or beautifully. This old man moved as if he had no bones.

I realized that after all my years of study, I still hadn't learned how to move; but, thank God, I had an idea of what I was supposed to do. We practiced for thirty minutes; he kept looking back at me to see if I'd tire out while he sunk lower and lower in his movements.

After we finished the form, he laughed and beckoned me to do "push hands" with him. Now, push hands is a T'ai Chi exercise usually done with two people. It uses basic techniques: ward-off, *P'eng;* roll-back, *Lu;* press, *Chi;* and push, *An.* The principles in push hands are the same as those in the solo exercise. However, more emphasis is placed on redirecting and neutralizing the external forces coming from the other person. I was amazed. His skin was as soft as a baby's, his muscles were completely relaxed and his fingertips glowed fire-red and his eyes glimmered. We touched hands. I felt something I had never experienced before, no bones. No bones! I am sure that if I ever shook the hand of a dragon it would feel exactly like that, no bones.

We began to do the push hands exercise of T'ai Chi Ch'uan, but when I began to push towards him, he "wasn't there" anymore. I felt nothing, no bones, no hands, no Tsao Li Ming. He seemed to disappear from my touch. All of a sudden, in the midst of a very slow circling movement, I lost my balance and was lifted up slightly off the ground. As I went back, I thought I'd try and see if I could get the old man. I didn't. To this day, I never have.

We pushed hands for about five minutes, after which I thanked him and smiled. He smiled back, throwing his hands up in the air and shrugging his shoulders as if to say, "That's it. That's how we should practice!"

He urged me to continue, but I didn't begin to study with him until a year later. I worked steadily with Tsao Li Ming for about seven months until he moved to San Francisco. However, we continued to keep in contact with one another.

On one of his visits to Chicago, I went to see him at his son's home. We started our conversation sociably over a cup of jasmine tea. Inevitably, we got into a conversation of T'ai Chi theory, covering everything from the basic principles through the martial arts, even into the Theory of Alchemy. Finally we decided to "play" T'ai Chi Ch'uan. He put on his Chinese shoes and we went into the basement so as to be undisturbed.

We went through the form together, I one step behind him, one moment behind, always, nonetheless, behind him. As we went through a posture called "snake creeps down," I saw his balance waiver, just sightly, but waiver. I'd never seen this before and wondered if maybe it wasn't the ground that moved since the old man never moved anywhere without being rooted. In my mind I began to question his strength. Once again I would try to uproot him, for I had become stronger and I did see him waiver. I began to get confident. I knew I could get him.

We started doing push hands. I had to be as soft as I could to gain a good position in our contest. So I reached down deep, down to the very core of my being for every last ounce of strength to become as soft as I could be. For the first time while dong push hands with Tsao Li Ming, it worked! For the next ten minutes I found myself neutralizing the old man's offense. Then, without a word between us, we both stopped. Although I did not uproot him, it was the first time the old man did not uproot me.

I was ecstatic, as I saw the old man walk away, he began to look very, very distant. The basement certainly couldn't be that long! Then he was gone. He seemed to disappear, then, he was right next to me at my left side. His left hand pushed directly on my face, his right hand at my stomach. A stream of air rushed between his hands and my body, I was pushed back, there he was in front of me smiling and uttering that curious laugh, "Ehhhh."

We never spoke much, but we both laughed a lot and there was lots of laughter even after this had occurred. He had gotten me again and this time with the style of a dragon pouncing on its prey.

The time I spent with Huo Chi Kwan made one hour seem like a cosmic eternity; whereas one hour with Tsao Li Ming felt like a cosmic flash, infinitesimally brief. In all of them, when Huo was Yang, Tsao was Yin; when Tsao was Yang, Huo was Yin. Huo was the tiger, Tsao the dragon.

Mr. Tsoi

During the time of my adventures with the tiger and the dragon, it was inevitable that I would encounter a Buddha on the path. Buddhas always travel incognito, but you can never miss them. They have two distinct characteristics, a round belly and a light in their eyes. The old Buddhist adage, "If you meet the Buddha, kill the Buddha" never made sense to me. Yet, this is the lesson I would learn from my friend Tsoi.

He was a man between medium and stocky build and 5'7" in height. He had a round, radiant face and his features and mannerisms made him look like the Chinese Humphrey Bogart. I'm sure he'd say that Humphrey Bogart was the American Mr. Tsoi.

His clothes were always crisp and neat, almost as if they were painted on. He always wore a bow tie. His basic beliefs were quite simple: don't believe anything, don't trust anyone and if you're about to get into a fight, hit first and ask questions later.

I first met this "old man" in 1968. I sensed he was a martial artist and he sensed I was, but it took two years before we started to talk. He was very impressed that I always said "thank you," "please," and "you're welcome." Good manners and politeness were of paramount importance to him. People without good manners angered him.

He got angry often. As I got to know him better through the years, I began to perceive his anger as humorous. In fact, it was comic. The angrier he got, the funnier he seemed. Of course, I never let him know that I perceived him this way, as I'm sure he wanted to show me how funny people look when they get angry.

Many times he came up to the table at the restaurant where he worked and mumbled a complaint about another waiter, customer, or as usually the case, his boss. As soon as he uttered the complaint, his entire countenance would change. He would become furious, but silent. As he walked away, I would start to laugh. Then he would proceed to treat all of the customers in a manner that fit his particular mood and I would laugh all the more as he silenced his emotions and anger.

Tsoi was a chronic gambler, addicted to the horses. That was no secret. He often lectured to me for what seemed to be hours on the evils of horse racing and gambling. Yet, every Monday Tsoi would

7

be at the track. By the end of the day he'd be tearing up his tickets, getting very angry. The next time I would see him he would complain about how he lost his entire week's wages on the horses. He claims to have lost several fortunes there and I sincerely believe he was serious about that. He gave the impression that he was at war with the racetrack owners and his job was to get all their money so no one else would lose at the track. Tsoi would bet against insurmountable odds. He feared nothing and he quite often lost. But somehow, in his immutable way, he always appeared the winner.

I never actually had classes with Mr. Tsoi. I never fought with him, and to this day, I can't remember his first name, though I know he showed it to me one day on his ID card. He was one of the few people I knew who could translate obscure phrases in classical Chinese. His martial art postures were clear and classical as though they had been set in place by a carpenter's rule.

On one occasion I recall him walking into the kitchen of the restaurant. Usually he would carry a platter over his head with one hand, kick the door with his foot, then walk through with flowing continuity. However, this time as he kicked open the door he made a curious circle with his left hand, forming a fist. This particular technique was something I'd been trying to learn for years. It was an integral part of certain T'ai Chi postures. Somehow, watching him do it unraveled the mysteries of the form.

Tsoi, like many Chinese martial artists, was studied in the theories of Chinese medicine. He spent eleven years in a monastery somewhere in southern China. There he learned various external and internal systems. Though he claimed to be a hard stylist, he did everything softly, effortlessly, and without tension. He was one of the most relaxed men I ever met, even when he was angry. That is one reason he seemed so funny.

Often when he spoke, he would transfer weight from one leg to another, giving the appearance of a slight sway. After watching him for two or three minutes, it looked as if the whole room was swaying with him.

Along with his trips to the racetrack, he was a fan of Bruce Lee and Kung Fu movies. Of course, he found time to practice daily, and from the looks of him, diligently.

Even though he wasn't a practitioner of T'ai Chi Ch'uan, he influenced my T'ai Chi Ch'uan greatly. Yet, the influence was much more than just movement or form. It was one of attitude, the attitude that all knowledge is within us all and that for a man to be free he must have no master, even if the Master is a Buddha.

I frequented the restaurant where Tsoi worked at least two or three times a week for seven years. Then, one day he disappeared and I never saw him again. To this day I still peer in the window of that restaurant to see if my old friend Tsoi is there. I often hear his voice as if he is whistling in the wind, whistling contently from a very distant land, a barren land where he has become content with himself. So he whistles and the land is filled with sound.

Tohei Sensei

Even in a barren land there can be many Buddhas, and it surprises me that some old Zen Master never coined the adage. "Once a Buddha, always a Buddha."

I spent very little time with Tohei Sensei. Although many T'ai Chi Ch'uan enthusiasts become so snooty that they won't accept the greatness of someone outside their art, I have seen none stand before this man. Professor Tohei's four basic principles, and all the principles he utilizes in teaching *Shinshin Toitsu Aikido* (Aikido with mind and body coordinated,) are essentially the same as those used in the T'ai Chi Ch'uan Classics.

Koichi Tohei came to Chicago often and every time he did I attended his seminars, often taking my students with me. On one occasion I recall him touching me on the side of the neck, softly and gently with three fingers. I lost consciousness. The next thing I recall, I was lying on the mat about ten feet away. My students later told me that he lifted me up off the ground about three feet and threw me back through the air a distance of about ten feet. All I can remember is his three fingers touching me on the side of the neck and hitting the mat very softly.

Koichi Tohei was born in 1920 and though he may fit into the category of an old man by many definitions, he's the youngest person I ever met. Certainly, he is one of the most charming. So charming, in fact, that when he smiles the gold crowns in his mouth sparkle giving the impression of sun beams shooting off in different directions from a distant star.

Most people, including myself, who have spent time on the mat with Tohei Sensei, envision him as a big man. He looks to be about 5'9" tall and sometimes 7' tall. He seems to weigh somewhere between 190 and 2,000 pounds. In fact, he is about 5'3" tall at most and as far as weight is concerned, it falls somewhere between the weights I mentioned.

Professor Tohei and I eventually became very good friends. On one occasion we went to lunch at a French restaurant in Chicago. After some wine and cocktails, we began to talk about martial arts in general. I should mention that there is another style of Aikido, taught by Kisshomaru Ueshiba who is the son of the founder of Aikido, Morihei Ueshiba. The elder Ueshiba is one of Professor Tohei's teachers. The younger Ueshiba and Tohei differ in their approaches. As a result, the Ueshiba camp, in typical Samurai fashion, is very critical of Tohei, for they believe that no one can teach Ki (Chi). Being able to teach Ki is the essential component of Tohei's philosophy.

Back at the luncheon, I informed Tohei Sensei that I attended a lecture given by a ninth degree Black Belt representative of the Ueshiba style and that he was most emphatic about the fact that no one can teach Ki. I believed it was directed particularly at Tohei's philosophy. Tohei responded very agreeably, shook his head almost sheepishly and said, "That's right. No one can teach Ki." He then bounded up smiling, gold crowns sparkling, looked me straight in the eye and continued, "Except me!"

Tohei's style of teaching was incredible. I have never seen anyone hold the attention of an audience and command their respect like Tohei. Going to his seminars was like attending the live performance of a rock and roll star. His dialogue was reminiscent of a great comedy. The expositions were dramatic, surrounded by tragedy, with an ironic, if not comic twist for an end, yet always happy, always laughing. You were constantly entertained as you learned.

If anything, Tohei's classes are infamous for their slapstick humor. Tohei often played the part of a disgruntled, grouchy, and egocentric person, often stomping on the floor, growling and insulting everyone and everything. Everyone would be in hysterics, and I'm sure they identified with many aspects of the character who resembled a Samurai Ebeneezer Scrooge.

This type of behavior, he would inform everyone, is not the right way and to develop Ki it is very important to develop good character. I once asked Tohei, "Why do you want to develop Ki?" He responded, "To develop good character." He also reminded me that using Ki is like using a sword. It could be used for good or evil.

Ch'i Development

If the road to hell is paved with good intentions,
the road to heaven is paved with Ch'i.

Chi cannot always fit within the bounds of human logic and is therefore undefinable. Any limitations on the word negate its definition. It has no definition nor any limitation. If Chi is beginning to sound like the ancient Chinese philosopher Lao Tsu's notion of the Tao, then incredibly, we are still too limited. It is much more than this, for every ancient culture revered the universal principle of Chi. "Chi" is a Chinese word. The Japanese call it "Ki," in Sanskrit it is "Prana," to the Greeks it was "Pneuma," to the Romans "Spiritus," in Hebrew "Ruakh," and for the Egyptians "Ka."

When you read the Bible in the original Greek, the term "Agion Pneuma" refers to the Holy Spirit, the breath of God. Chi, and its cultural equivalents in other ancient languages, could mean far more: the sustaining principle of life in the whole universe, the life force, internal energy, our breath, the electrical pulsations of our nervous systems. It is the Universal Chi that acts in us through love, understanding, compassion, sincerity, truth, and justice. It is the Universal Chi that sustains life.

Chi is free, but it is a pearl of great price. We all have it, but very few of us find it. We all see it, but very few of us know it is there. We all hear it, but very few of us listen. We all want it, but very few of us get it.

Einstein showed with his theory of relativity that matter and energy are equatable and differ only by a numerical constant, $E = mc^2$.

11

Scientists, in understanding part of the vast implications of this theory, took matter in the form of uranium and transformed it into our first atomic bomb, energy. Now we have nuclear power plants all over. Yet, it is readily apparent even to a layman, that if with our primitive capacities we can transform matter into energy and energy into matter, the probabilities for future transformations are endless.

Chi is energy, but it is also more than energy. It is also matter, animate and inanimate. We should realize the different forms that energy can assume. As human beings we are concerned with the transformation and realization of our own energy, our Chi and matter, just as scientists realized the awesome strength found in a naturally occurring element. This is the Chi development, the Chi Kung of T'ai Chi. It is the essence of the art, the cultivation of not only our personal life force, but harmony with the Universal Life Force. This is T'ai Chi.

In T'ai Chi we subscribe to the Chi theory, not on faith or belief alone, but in understanding. To have this understanding, we must eliminate doubt.

Though faith and belief are important to each human being, the words "faith" and "belief" imply that there is not a total understanding. To believe is not necessarily to know. To have understanding means to know while eliminating all doubts. In T'ai Chi understanding comes as a personal experience. Therefore, T'ai Chi is often considered to be personalized in form.

There are many approaches for developing the Chi, but we will discuss only four of them.

Breath

The most common technique for Chi development in T'ai Chi Ch'uan is through the coordination of breath and movement. Each and every move is totally correlated with a well-defined breathing pattern that integrates form and movement. Most T'ai Chi books attempt to explain this in the simple terms of expansion and contraction, opening and closing, raising and lowering. However, these are only general guides since they can not completely integrate the breath with each part of the form, nor with the whole of the form itself.

There are two components within each breath, Yin and Yang, inhale and exhale. In T'ai Chi, "our emphasis lies not in the movement of form, but in the movement and coordination of breath; not in external aspects, but in the internal situation; not in the physical form, but in the breath that guides the form." The student understands breath in terms of form. The teacher understands breath in terms of Breath.

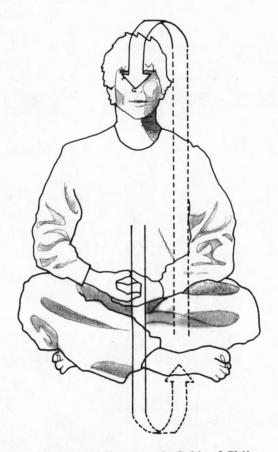

Figure 1: Microcosmic Orbit of Ch'i

Tsao Li Ming's approach to T'ai Chi Ch'uan was wholly intertwined with the processes of Taoist Yoga and that of alchemy, or transubstantiation. Often before practicing he would sit quietly on the ground or a chair and practice a breathing exercise known in T'ai Chi as the microcosmic orbit. It is depicted in more detail in the diagram above. (For other diagrams, see Wen Shang Huang's work, *Fundamentals of T'ai Chi Ch'uan*.)

During other sessions, Tsao would stand erect and practice what is known as the macrocosmic orbit, first on the right side, and then on the left.

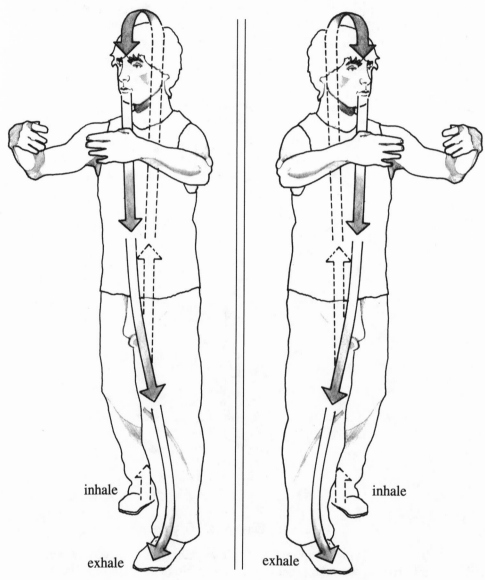

inhale

exhale

inhale

exhale

Figure 2: Macrocosmic Orbit of Chi

Although these auxilliary breathing exercises are both useful and effective, it is within the T'ai Chi Ch'uan exercise itself that the true cultivation of Chi and breath is at its zenith; movement and breath in harmonious oneness.

Mind/Body Coordination

Today some cults and occult practices are aimed at separating mind and body: astral projection, hallucinogens, and certain types of yoga are all examples of this. For those who wish to do this, I can recommend a very simple and very effective way to separate mind and body: Die!

If we want to be healthy human beings, it is a good idea to coordinate mind and body. These other techniques that serve to separate mind and body often do so because they consider the body inferior to the mind. In T'ai Chi we are not concerned with the issue of superiority. We have a mind and we have a body and we feel much better when they are working in harmony.

The simplest approach to mind/body coordination is that taught by Koichi Tohei. He often relates the story of a Karate instructor who invited him to his office. As the instructor sat behind his desk, he pulled out a bottle of ink and placed it on the desk. He stared at the bottle very intensely with a long, drawn face. He continued to stare at it harder and harder, deeper and deeper, until Professor Tohei asked him what he was doing. The Karate instructor replied, "I am trying to use my Ki to move the ink bottle." Tohei asked, "Any success?" The Karate instructor retorted in a very low gruff voice, "Not yet." Then he looked at Tohei and asked, "Can you do it, Teacher?" Tohei responded, "Certainly I can!" He then promptly extended his arm, grabbed the ink bottle and brought it across the desk to the Karate instructor's amazement. The instructor complained, "That's not fair. You used your arm." Professor Tohei calmly responded: "But I used my Ki to move my arm!"

Tohei's method of teaching Chi development with mind/body coordination utilizes four basic principles. These principles are indeed one in the same and are all different ways of looking at a singular truth. They are: (1) Keep one-point; (2) Relax completely; (3) Keep weight underside; and (4) Extend Ki.

Keeping One-Point

To someone who doesn't grasp English translations of Japanese concepts, the principles as stated make no sense at all. It's not the words that are important, but the feeling, and the feeling is universal. To keep one-point means that your mind is focused on your "one-point," the single point that lies two to three inches below the navel and which conspicuously accords with your center of mass. In T'ai Chi we may refer to this as our *Tan Tien.* It is not a question of finding the Tan Tien, but the feeling you get when the mind is focused on Tan Tien. "Tan Tien" translated into English means "Sea of Cinnabar." Hence, the Chinese term does not refer solely to the single point which Tohei refers to as the one-point, but also to the entire region which the Japanese refer to as "Hara."

Keeping one-point means centering, focusing, or even concentrating one's mind on the point of mind and body just below the navel. Remember, centering implies more than just balance. Keeping one-point and centering include the notion of balance and much more. It is a focused balance, a unified balance, a well-defined balance, a concentrated balance. It is a stabilizing effect on one's whole being. Keeping the mind centered on the one-point automatically unifies the mind and body. The whole of the Universe pours into the one point.

In acupuncture theory, Tan Tien falls within the meridian points at the back of the body labeled Governing Vessel 3, 4, and 5. Corresponding points on the front of the body are Conception Vessel 5, 6, and 7. There is disagreement on the question of which of these acupuncture points in fact correspond to the one-point, if any of them do. In any case, to keep one-point is to unify mind and body. To keep one-point is to exercise and develop the Chi.

Relax Completely

The idea of relaxing completely emphasizes "completely." To be complete, each and every muscle and joint must be relaxed. The mind must be equally calm. In this sense, if relaxation is not complete it is not relaxation. The Chinese term "Sung" encompasses the idea of complete relaxation. In fact, Tohei's English expression "Relax Completely" is identical to the Chinese term Sung.

16

It is interesting to note that there is great difficulty in translating the concept Sung into English. The Chinese character for Sung is compressed from many smaller characters. Etymologically, Sung means "hairy pine tree." Now, it would be very easy to be mysterious and say that T'ai Chi is like a hairy pine tree. Instead, let's consider the word Sung to be relaxation, looseness, softness, buoyancy, resiliency, and suppleness all put together. My good friend George Lee calls it looseness relaxation.

Keep Weight Underside

Keeping weight underside means to not fight gravity and let your weight follow its natural course downward. If we lift our arm, for example, we shouldn't use our arm and shoulder muscles to resist gravity. Rather, use the muscles just enough to lift the arm while keeping the weight of the arm down. That is, the weight is in the underside of the arm.

Keeping the weight underside, though, does not mean surrendering to gravity, for then we would fall down. It means not to resist gravity.

There is a fine line between not resisting and surrendering that can be bridged if we consider the notion of sinking. As you lift your arm up its weight should naturally sink down. Your entire body must also be felt to be sinking its weight down to the ground. Analogously, your breathing should be low and diaphragmatic. Thus, keeping weight underside means letting your weight sink down naturally and continuously.

Extend Ki

To extend Ki or Chi means to direct your energy and spirit outwards. If you keep one-point, relax completely and have weight underside, you will naturally focus and direct your energies outward. Extending Chi allows us to have awareness not only of ourselves, but also of that which is around us. It is the natural flow of one's energy outward, unimpeded, unobstructed, and continuous. Without the notion of extending, we cannot love or understand other people. It is a vitalization of mind and body that serves to coordinate mind and body.

17

If we consider the question, "Why is the Dead Sea dead?", we will understand why we need to follow this principle always. The Dead Sea is dead because it only has tributaries leading in and none leading out. To extend our Chi means to replenish it.

We can see that keeping one-point and extending Chi are rules of mind that unify mind and body. To relax completely and keep weight underside are rules of the body that coordinate mind and body. In fact, they are each different facets of Chi development and mind/body unification. Thus, if you attain one you attain them all. If you lose one, you lose them all.

Meditation

Let us "meditate" on meditation. The idea of meditation contains the mental ingredients of calmness, stillness, union, peace, harmony, and the concentration of mental powers. But to try to define the situation known as meditation would annihilate it. "Annihilate" is a good word because it is more final than ending or destroying. To annihilate is to remove from reality and meditation must make us aware of reality.

Reality is such a wonderful thing. It is so wonderful that it has no opposite in the universe. We can think about what's not real, but it will still not be real. Meditation is a union, a yoga if you will, since the Sanskrit word "yoga" means union or yoking. What are we yoked to? The answer, of course, is nothing and therefore we have a union with the whole.

Some cults fabricate a notion of the mysterious, the cosmic, the esoteric, when presenting meditation. Meditation has nothing to do with cults, although cults have fed on the idea like leeches. Once a group has incorporated their exclusive type of meditation by which they try to corner the market on truth, they have created a wall and it is this wall that excludes them from the whole.

This wall is their illusion and their illusion leads to annihilation. Therefore, the goal of meditation lies not in the technique, because there are many good techniques. Rather, meditation is in the situation and in the perpetuation of the mental practices that give us a healthy mind. The meditative mind is a meditative mind twenty-four hours a day. It cannot be described in the irregular and erratic behaviors that characterize the neurotic man. Nor is it visible in the zombie mind that is found in many cults. It is the Real mind and thus, the Real Man or Woman.

Any time you obtain this meditative frame of mind with all the ingredients I have mentioned, the serene composure of mind affects the body and your natural energy flows unimpeded. If the body is unrefined mind and the mind refined body, then the technique of meditation further refines both.

There is nothing mysterious or occult in meditation. It is our natural state. It is state of rapture, yet, it leads to ultimate awareness and totally transcends the conscious and subconscious mind. The walls between the conscious and subconscious mind break down. There is no separation.

As a technique, one needn't sit in a lotus posture unless one feels inclined to do so. One can meditate sitting down, lying down, standing up, running, walking, whirling around, sleeping, or any time at all. If you look around you and calmly observe life and your surroundings, this is also a meditation. But to quiet the mind is not a trivial endeavor. One must not resist any thought that comes into the mind, good or ill. Yet, neither should we be attached or hang on to them.

To meditate is also to reflect. Although meditation is a state, it is also an exercise in attaining that state. To attain the state, we must exercise the state. For most modern men who cannot maintain peace of mind, there is then a need to exercise the mind through meditation. The whole of T'ai Chi Ch'uan is a meditative exercise.

Physical Exercise

Anyone who does physical exercise of any kind will strengthen their vitality and spirit. Generally, people who exercise regularly are more full of life, more vibrant, and more at ease than those who do not. They have improved their physical condition and this automatically improves the mind. This is, indeed, the ancient Greek notion of sound mind and sound body. We see that any kind of physical exercise, especially when done regularly, develops the Chi. It was a natural step for man to design exercises that would specifically and effectively develop the Chi.

In T'ai Chi Ch'uan, Hatha Yoga, Aikido, and other Chi development exercise, the physical conditioning is geared to maximize Chi development. One must develop the T'ai Chi body. To develop the T'ai Chi body is to be like a child with all of the agility, suppleness, softness, and tenacious energy associated with a child. It is only then that the inner organs will work completely and harmoniously, that the circulation of the blood will be free and unobstructed, that the breathing will be soft, low, and dynamic, that the joints open up and the muscles become supple and pliable, and that the bones have the suppleness and strength of refined steel. It is only then, when we become like children again, that the Chi takes its useful course in the body.

T'ai Chi Ch'uan is a very powerful tool in this regard. In developing our Chi we must immediately use it in good ways and with good means.

The Theory of
T'ai Chi Ch'uan

Treat the Chi as the guest; it is not the host.
Don't be afraid of losing yourself in heaven.
The great tide is not like a droplet lost in a
great ocean, for it is the ocean that comes in
to fill the droplet.

The solo exercise is the heart of T'ai Chi Ch'uan. It is both simple and complex, hard and soft, sinking as well as rising. The daily practice of the solo exercise awakens the Chi. The Chi, in turn, develops the Chin, the internal power of the T'ai Chi body, and together they awaken the mind. When the mind awakens, the body follows, all things according to their own nature.

If we compare our bodies to a steam engine, the Chi would be analogous to the steam necessary to produce the power to drive the engine. The power developed in the engine would be analogous to the Chin. The Chin, the internal power of the body, embraces two characteristics, resilient flexibility, and bouncy suppleness. In our own bodies, when the Chi sinks down, the Chin lifts up, though the essential nature of the Chin is like that of mercury in that it both sinks and flows swiftly. The power of Chin often feels like an internal vibration; as the vibration becomes faster and faster, the Chin becomes more powerful.

The solo exercise is designed to exercise the body, strengthen the mind, awaken the Chi, and develop the Chin. For the most part our Chi is inherent; we are born with it. The purpose of Chi development is two-fold. First, we must awaken, focus, and direct what Chi we were born with, our primal Chi. Next, we must further develop and increase what we already have. But in the case of the Chin, it must be developed.

21

In performing the solo exercise, we follow certain principles. We learn these principles to be correct through our personal experience. For example, we all understand that being relaxed feels better than being tense. We will consider nine essential principles of T'ai Chi. Before doing this, however, we must first understand what is meant by correct posture. Once we maintain correct posture we may use the basic principles as the dynamics of T'ai Chi and its movement.

Posture

T'ai Chi is an art of movement and its dynamics distinguish it from other forms of exercise. Correct posture and excellence of movement are inseparable in T'ai Chi. The basic principles of posture are:

- Suppose your head is hung from a string.
- Look forward.
- Close your mouth.
- Touch your tongue to the roof of your mouth.
- Breathe through your nose, naturally.
- Relax mind and body.
- Keep your head and spine aligned.
- Keep the weight of your shoulders and elbows down.

These basic principles of posture must be maintained throughout the practice of all T'ai Chi exercise. If not kept, the movement will be wrong. Let's examine the components of T'ai Chi movement.

Relaxation

Relaxation is the fundamental guiding principle of T'ai Chi. The entire body must be relaxed always. But what is meant by relaxation? It is, of course, freedom from tension and strain. The body is light, supple, and at ease. However, relaxation is not letting the body go limp or lazy. Very often beginning students make this mistake and let the body hang like a piece of dead meat. In T'ai Chi, relaxation is alive and vital, while at the same time comfortable and at ease.

To acquire complete relaxation of the body, we must first calm the mind. Before you begin moving you must stand quietly for several minutes until you feel the entire body at ease and composed. All systems of T'ai Chi incorporate this time of preparation. If disturbing thoughts come, don't fight. Let them come, but don't hold on to them. Let them go. As the mind becomes really calm, you will feel it in your body. Now and only now can you begin to move correctly. This state of mind is not erratic or jumpy, but calm and serene. On the other hand, it is not a trance-like or hypnotic frame of mind; rather, alive, alert, and aware.

If a muscle or joint becomes tense, let it go. Consciously relax the muscle and release the tenseness. Relaxation in T'ai Chi is expressed through the term "Sung." Sung implies relaxation, looseness, sinking and vitality. In T'ai Chi, to relax is to seek serenity in the midst of activity and know the active through the passive. Sung is complete. The body feels almost transparent and porous as if air can circulate through and permeate the entire body. The body begins to feel as if there were no bones, or at least that the bones are extremely resilient.

Harmony

Calming the mind and relaxing the body result in the coordination of mind and body. The harmony of mind and body produces harmony of movement. When one of the muscles or joints move all the other muscles and joints move in coordination. At first the beginner pays attention to the coordination of arms and legs. There is no independent arm movement. Arms and legs move in an integrated mobility. Thus, we can coordinate the shoulders and inner thighs, the elbows and knees, and the hands and feet. These are termed the three external coordinations. The three internal coordinations are the will and the mind, the mind and the Chi and the Chi and the body.

Classically, it is said that the joints should feel as if they were strung together like pearls on a string. Attaining this complete harmony of motion is not a trivial matter. The key lies in the movement of the waist. It is the waist that coordinates all the different parts of the body. In fact, the waist directs all movement. Yet, it is the mind that directs the waist motion through the Chi. Subsequently, the waist motion directs the movement of the body.

Paradoxically, when you wish to move to the right you must first turn slightly to the left. If you wish to move forward, first withdraw slightly. If you wish to move upward, first sink slightly down. This complementary motion develops fluidity, balance, and continuity of motion. But there should be a clear distinction between the waist and the hips, to avoid losing the center of gravity which is kept firmly over the weighted leg. When the waist moves, the hips do not necessarily turn very much. The knees move even less and should never be allowed to collapse and lose the dynamics of a rooted stance.

Differentiation

In T'ai Chi, differentiation is the ability to separate. The principles of differentiation and harmony are paradoxically not in opposition. It is only by knowing the polarity of Yin and Yang that we can blend them to achieve the harmony of T'ai Chi. When Yang is substantial, Yin is insubstantial. When Yang is plus, Yin is minus. If Yang is active, Yin becomes passive. Yin and Yang are mutually exclusive categories like hot and cold, male and female, light and dark, day and night, and so forth. When Yin and Yang are in harmony, we have T'ai Chi. This is called the theory of complementary opposites.

Generally, in classical T'ai Chi the leg that sustains most or all the body weight is termed Yang. The leg that holds up little or no weight is called Yin. As in physics, when we create a potential difference, a current will begin to flow. This is how we create the electricity that lights our homes. In our T'ai Chi movement, the potential difference created by the differentiation of Yin and Yang produces the current of Chi that flows through our nervous system. Furthermore, according to the theory of Yin and Yang, if our right leg is Yang, our left arm is Yang. If our left leg is Yang, our right arm is Yang. This is another differentiation according to the theory of complementary opposites.

Now a pedantic reader might say that as we move and transfer our weight from one leg to another, there will be a single point when we will be double-weighted, having fifty percent of our body weight on each leg. This would apparently violate the principle of differentiation. But, if our movement is continuous as it must be in all of our T'ai Chi movements, then we would be double-weighted only at a single point in time. There being no time interval in a single point, our continuous motion would maintain the principle of differentiation.

Since all classical T'ai Chi exercises begin and end with the weight being equally distributed on both feet, it seems as if we would once again violate our rule for differentiating the substantial from the insubstantial. However, for these two stationary postures, the commencement and conclusion of the solo exercise, we may consider the lower torso Yang and the upper torso Yin. Furthermore when we begin (or complete) the solo exercises, one side of the body becomes Yang and the other Yin.

To be in accord with the principle of harmony, the well-blended differentiation of Yin and Yang is the harmony of T'ai Chi. What is by nature Yang is Yang. What is by nature Yin is Yin. Yet we note that within the Yang there is an element of Yin and within the Yin there is an element of Yang. This indeed does not change the nature of Yin and Yang but serves to better define and allow for the T'ai Chi harmony.

Centering

If our T'ai Chi is to be relaxed and harmonious, we must feel secure in our postures. This is the basis of centering. Centering is just as much a matter of mind as it is of the body. Centering is more than just balance; it includes balance and much more. If in the context of our T'ai Chi practice we perform a posture standing on one leg, we may be balanced, but a strong gust of wind or a slight push would up-end us. When one is truly centered, this does not happen.

Focusing the mind to the Tan Tien and concentrating the Tan Tien to a single point two to three inches below the navel is the basis of centering. It is a point of mind and may have no physiological counterpart. By focusing and concentrating in a relaxed and natural manner, we are more aware of our bodies and everything around us. Relaxation, harmony, and centering are inseparable components of T'ai Chi. If you achieve one, you achieve all three and if you fail at one, you fail at the others.

Recall that the center of gravity must rest upon the weighted leg. When you shift the weight to the opposite leg, make sure the center of gravity is firmly rooted on one leg before you move your weight or your transition will not be secure and centered. Furthermore, the transfer must be smooth and continuous. Any instability is due to double-weightedness; that is, allowing the weight to be equally distributed on both legs for any interval of time during movement. It is sometimes easier for beginners to incline the upper body just slightly while maintaining the head and spine straight. Classically, this involves the alignment of the Tan Tien with the Ming Tang, or the point of reference just above the nose and between the eyes. Centering, however, must be maintained at any angle or inclination.

Circularity

All T'ai Chi movements are circular, spiral, or in the form of arches or circles. As you progress, you will add circles to the movement; from big circles to small circles, to circles within circles, and finally invisible circles. Avoid straight and flat movement. Circularity is an essential character of T'ai Chi. Besides circularity of motion, the limbs must maintain a curvature. The classics refer to this as the "curved seeking straightness." Never lock the knees, elbows, or any joint in a straight line. This not only affects the fluidity of your motion, but impedes the natural flow of the Chi through the body.

Consider the "five bows" of T'ai Chi Ch'uan. Keeping the elbows bent, with shoulders and wrists relaxed, is termed the "bows of the arms." Keeping the knees slightly bent, hips and ankles relaxed, is the "bows of the legs." It is beneficial if the knees do not extend over the toes, since this makes it difficult for the center of gravity to rest naturally over the weighted leg. When standing on one leg, maintain a slight bend in the knee or the body will not feel secure.

Finally, the "bow of the body" refers to flexible, springlike resiliency of the spine. Keep the head and spine on one line, yet flexible and springlike as you move. The rotating motion of the waist around the aligned and resilient spine massages and tonifies the internal organs. This action is fundamental in acquiring the benefits of T'ai Chi for the health of the inner organs. There is no other exercise that emphasizes this action in its entirety. In time, the tonification and strengthening of all internal organs strengthens and tonifies the entire body.

Continuity

The end of one T'ai Chi posture is the beginning of the next. Each and every movement must be brought to its completion with the movements clearly defined and not run together. There are no gaps or pauses at any time and the continuity of motion is free-flowing while integrating every part of the body. Most important is continuity of the extension and flow of the Chi. This brings us to a point often neglected not only by beginners but by teachers of the art as well.

The Classics point out that T'ai Chi is concerned with storing energy as well as releasing energy. The key to the continuous flow of Chi as well as continuity of movement is to extend the Chi. Extending one's Chi means to allow our natural and intrinsic energy to flow outward at all times. To try to store up all our Chi would be like developing power in a machine that has no outlet. The machine would inevitably burn up. Likewise, in a reservoir of water that has no natural outlet, the water stagnates. Throughout our practice of T'ai Chi we must, with our minds, let the Chi extend naturally and continuously.

In T'ai Chi, continuity means more than just movement. Besides the idea of not stopping our movement and extension, motion must also be smooth, void of abruptness, pauses, or stops. The Classics poetically refer to the continuous motion of T'ai Chi as reeling silk from a cocoon. To prevent the thread of silk from breaking, it must be drawn out continuously and in smooth fashion. Because most of us have never reeled silk from a cocoon, it may be easier to consider the waves of the ocean. The waves rise and fall fluidly, continuously and smoothly, each one flowing into the other and connected by the water's motions.

Slowness

Another characteristic of T'ai Chi that differentiates it from most other forms of exercise is the principle of slowness. All movement should be slow. The effect of slowness is that the body begins to heat up without straining or overly perspiring and thus the joints begin to open up and the Chi flows unimpeded. Stretching the muscles will not by itself cause the joints to open. It is through slowness that we begin to feel the effects of the Chi and better command the Chi to move the body.

We should not, however, move so slowly as to make tension in the body. Generally, the slower the movement the better the movement is for developing the Chi. The beginning student must not only move slowly and smoothly, but maintain the same speed throughout the form, the pace of that day depending on one's condition.

Next, the student should develop a sense of rhythm. Etymologically, the word "rhythm" means flow. As the student develops an internal flow of Chi, a natural rhythm permeates the body and its motion. This natural rhythm creates movement and waves that cannot be mimicked by any muscular exertion. The body is virtually ethereal and floats like a cloud; at the same time, this rhythm creates a root with unlimited depth that creates the stability and

27

substantiality to harmonize the airy and insubstantial motion. This is T'ai Chi.

Rhythm comes out of slowness and accordance with all the other principles of T'ai Chi movement. Yet, it is only when the Chi circulates unimpeded through every part of the body that slowness can truly become rhythm. Rhythm, then, is the perfect blend of time and space. Each T'ai Chi posture must occupy the right space at the right time.

It should be noted that to insist that every movement must be done at the same speed throughout the solo exercise is only a first step. Yang Chang Fu and Wu Chien Ch'uan once gave a joint exhibition in China in the early part of this century. Their movement was described as being very soft and fluid, totally continuous, yet changing speed to fit the proper arc, curve, line, or single point. They did not do each and every movement at the same speed, but they did have a harmonious rhythm not only within their own movements, but also with respect to each other, even though they each demonstrated a different form.

Absolute Softness

The principle of absolute softness distinguishes T'ai Chi Ch'uan among all other martial arts. The softer and more supple your movement, the stronger and more sensitive your body becomes. Although this idea seems to be a paradox, it is readily observable in anyone who does T'ai Chi.

We have said that to be truly relaxed, one must be alive and aware and not limp like dead meat. Similarly, with softness the movement is alive and supple, but in accord with the theory of Yin and Yang. The state of softness is, in fact, hardness and softness well blended. By hardness we do not mean tensing the muscles, since this would violate the principle of relaxation. By hardness we mean relaxed and supple movement, not lazy and void of life. Thus, in T'ai Chi we are soft, but not to the point of collapse; and hard, but not to the point of rigidity. Consider a water hose where water rushing through gives the hose hardness while the hose remains supple.

As a general order of training common to all styles of T'ai Chi Ch'uan, the student progresses from softness to hardness, from hardness back to softness again and finally, hardness and softness well blended, T'ai Chi, "wonderful hand of air." After a few years of practice the entire body feels like cotton wrapped around iron, internally very firm while externally very supple. Sometimes during the practice of T'ai Chi, the beginner may feel the bones and joints becoming steel-hard without effort. The Classics refer to the Chi permeating to the very marrow of the bone. This is indeed a high level of achievement, but by no means an end.

Sinking

In the Classics, "sinking the Chi to the Tan Tien" is the root of internal development. First of all this means that our breathing should be diaphragmatic. When we inhale our lungs fill with air, pushing the diaphragm down and expanding the abdomen. When we exhale, the air comes out of the lungs, the diaphragm comes up and the abdomen contracts. Of course this breathing is natural and relaxed, while at the same time long and continuous. In short, the breathing is very similar to that of a child's. After a while, the expansion and contraction of the abdomen is undetectable and the breath is deep but silent.

Next, sinking the Chi to the Tan Tien refers to focusing the mind at the Tan Tien. Also it means that we should keep the weight of our bodies continuously going downward, going with and not fighting against gravity. Even if we extend our arms or legs upward, the weight of the arms or legs must be naturally underside down, in harmony with gravity.

Sinking also refers to the physical act of sinking at the culmination of a T'ai Chi posture. Besides the natural act of sinking, the entire body seems to expand and becomes a very heavy mass centered at one-point. Yet, in accordance with our principles, before there is sinking there should be a slight rise. Very often T'ai Chi teachers will tell their students to maintain the same height throughout the practice of T'ai Chi. Not only is this unnatural, it stifles the free flowing fluidity of the art.

As a final and most important note in sinking, consider the relation of sinking to centering. The coccyx and buttocks never stick out during your practice. Remember the importance of correct posture without which we cannot be truly centered or sinking in our movement.

To summarize the notion of sinking, we consider the Yueh Chun or "bubbling well" located near the center of the sole of the foot, at the first point of the Kidney Meridian. When we put together all the notions of sinking, the Chi is said to sink to the "bubbling

29

well." This means your center of gravity is at its lowest point. The body develops a powerful root to the ground and the whole body above this point has maximum resiliency. This is also the Yin and Yang of weight distribution for the feet. Always keeping the weight of the body at the "bubbling well" of the Yang leg is a good approach for beginners.

Summary

At first, you will have to think about doing these things. However, after a few months of daily practice the principles become instinctive and natural. This does not necessarily mean simple and easy, since we can always improve on what we have done. There is no perfection in T'ai Chi just as there are no limitations. It is a growing art: "When Yin and Yang are in harmony, ten thousand things grow." This is the essence of T'ai Chi Ch'uan.

Delineating the principles of posture, mind and body coordination, or T'ai Chi movement helps us to develop mind, body, and spirit. There are many things to think about. As a note of caution we must not become fixated or rigid in applying these terms. This is why Koichi Tohei says, in discussing concentration of the one-point (keeping one-point), to also be unconscious of your lower abdomen. (You cannot keep one-point if you are conscious only of your abdominal area.) In the case of aligning the head and spine, you must not rigidly position the spine or body without retaining pliability. In other words, don't get hung up on the words. All of this is a natural state and it is very difficult to erase years of unnatural habits in a short time. At first, some T'ai Chi postures may feel very unnatural. Yet the postures and movement are indeed natural. It is our bodies themselves that have taken on the unnatural development that expresses itself in hardness, rigidity, disease, and death. Disease and death are no more natural than rigidity and tension. To be natural is not a learned state, therefore much of T'ai Chi involves unlearning as well as learning.

The nine essential principles may be derived from four essential points: complete relaxation of the body; calmness of the mind; serenity of the Chi; and soft and supple movement. As we practice our T'ai Chi, we will naturally carry these principles into our daily lives. Therefore, the true practitioner of the art must practice twenty-four hours a day, without interruption, continuously and naturally.

Chi Kung

and the

Essential Movements of T'ai Chi Ch'uan

"The way of heaven is to benefit, not to harm."
— *Lao Tsu*

Chi Kung is the art of Chi development in the *Nei Kung,* or inner school of Chinese Physical Culture. Traditionally the old schools of T'ai Chi taught a series of eight basic postures that could be done singularly, or as a series of movements. These basic movements would form a foundation for other solo exercises, and were used to strengthen the body, stretch the muscles, open the joints, and begin the development of Chi. Thus, they were termed "Chi Kung," or Chi development exercises.

These exercises are seldom taught today because adapting T'ai Chi Ch'uan for the general public has required simplifying and relaxing many of the training methods. However, anyone who wishes to master a trade, an art, or a sport must have a firm foundation rooted in good basics. T'ai Chi Ch'uan requires a good foundation and continued emphasis on basics. Without this, the entire structure will be weak. The basics, then, are practiced not only by beginners, but also by advanced practitioners who wish to progress by strengthening their foundation.

Basics are difficult. Yet they are important because they are immediately derived from the basic principles. These basic exercises can be practiced by practitioners of the Chen, Yang, Wu, or any other style of T'ai Chi and can contribute by further opening the joints, stretching the sinews and ligaments, harmonizing the internal organs, calming and developing the Chi, and affecting the Chin. The principles of the basic movement of T'ai Chi Ch'uan are the same as those in all solo exercises. Although the differentiation of Yin and Yang may vary in structure, it is nonetheless there.

This set of exercises is best when done for twenty to forty minutes, after which the solo exercises can be practiced to a fuller degree. There are no short cuts in T'ai Chi Ch'uan. Transformation into the T'ai Chi body takes time. The basic movement is an exercise in time, as much as an exercise in movement.

Heaven
The Creative

The Preparation

"Great indeed is the generating power of the Creative.
All beings owe their beginning to it."
— *Confucius*

The Preparation is standing meditation. Mind, Body and Spirit become one. Many people skip over the Preparation. This is a big mistake. It is a complete "T'ai Chi." It is the simplest possible posture; you just stand there. Yet, to align the spine as it should be in the Preparation is a most difficult accomplishment.

Note the directives that accompany Figure 3 (next page). These principles must be maintained throughout the practice of T'ai Chi Ch'uan. Remain in this preparatory posture for as long as it takes to develop a relaxed body, calm mind, and serene outlook. Usually five minutes is sufficient, but take care that every muscle in the body is soft, supple and relaxed, yet at the same time alert, sensitive, and aware. Empty the weight of your upper torso down to the "bubbling well."

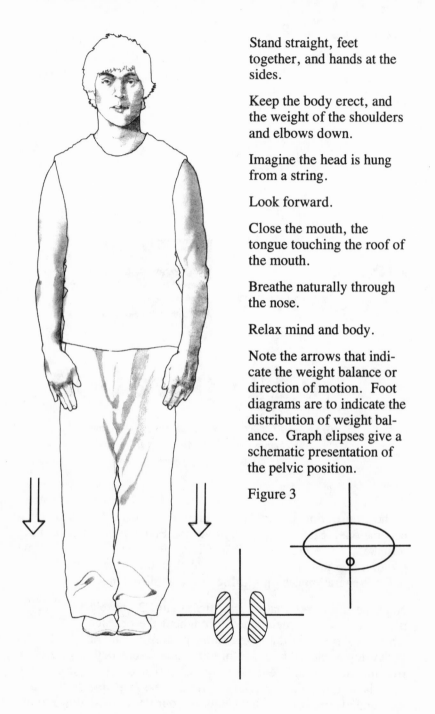

Stand straight, feet together, and hands at the sides.

Keep the body erect, and the weight of the shoulders and elbows down.

Imagine the head is hung from a string.

Look forward.

Close the mouth, the tongue touching the roof of the mouth.

Breathe naturally through the nose.

Relax mind and body.

Note the arrows that indicate the weight balance or direction of motion. Foot diagrams are to indicate the distribution of weight balance. Graph elipses give a schematic presentation of the pelvic position.

Figure 3

What is meant by supposing your head to be hung from a string is that the "lift" of this erect posture will let your body relax. You should immediately feel relaxation in the neck and shoulders as your muscles, joints, and bones fall into line.

As you look forward don't fix on any particular point, but don't stare blankly into space. Your vision is alert and relaxed. If you become overly intent on what you are looking at, close your eyes half way. If introspection is needed, you may close your eyes lightly.

The purpose of keeping the tongue in contact with the roof of the mouth and keeping the mouth closed is to form a connection between the Conception Vessel and Governing Vessel meridians. This completes a primary circulation of Chi energy called the Microcosmic Orbit. Furthermore, the saliva is activated and swallowed, not spit out, keeping the mouth and throat from becoming dry.

Remember not to force your breathing. Natural breathing is like a baby's, soft, relaxed, and from the diaphragm. Each inhale and each exhale should be complete and even.

Relaxing the body begins with relaxing your mind. The mind leads the body. This is difficult at first. Thoughts will come into your mind and you will tend to "fight them off." This will just concentrate your attention even more on the thought. Let your thoughts pass, don't hold on. Let your thoughts go by. If you need help, concentrate on relaxing, in turn, every muscle in your body. From the tips of your toes to the top of your head make sure there is no tension. Keep your fingertips pointing slightly down to help extend your Chi internally through the whole body.

Keeping your body erect means to align the spine so the vertebrae are straight, springlike, and open. At first you will have to concentrate to keep from sinking into a habitual slump.

Don't fight gravity. Let the weight of your torso empty into your legs and down into the bubbling well at the soles of your feet. This weight at the soles and heels stimulates the Kidney Meridian.

The key to this posture is the state of relaxation and serenity. Usually five minutes is enough. It is important that every muscle of your body become soft, supple, and relaxed. As the Chi begins to circulate each individual may begin to feel a variety of different feelings. You may experience your body heating up, or a feeling of energy in your feet or fingers, sometimes up the spine itself. Some people experience an intense tingling, like an electric charge or magnetic polarity. All these stimulations indicate the movement of Chi and the beginning of Chi cultivation. These are short term effects and in no more than a month and often right away, you will feel your body begin to change more.

Mountain
Keeping Still

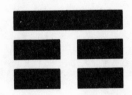

Holding the Ball

*"The superior man forsees all human concerns
and is not disturbed by any accident of fortune."*
— *Pythagoras*

Having done the Preparation for five minutes, or for as long as it takes to relax the body entirely and stimulate the flow of energy, you are ready to move on to the next movement called the Map of T'ai Chi or more simply Holding the Ball.

Like the Preparation, this is a static posture. However, the internal movement of Chi allows for the active within the inactive. After the Chi has begun to circulate in the Preparation, Holding the Ball develops a stronger circulation of Chi and can be likened to the charging of a battery. In T'ai Chi we are not only concerned with the stretching and pliability of the body, but also with elasticity and resiliency of the muscles themselves. T'ai Chi muscle tone is not only long, but resilient and dense.

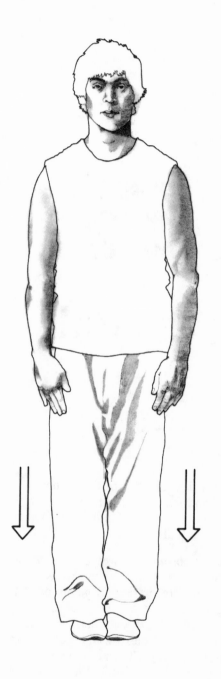

From the Preparation, sit a little by slightly bending both knees.

Figure 4

Place all your weight on the right foot and lift the left heel.

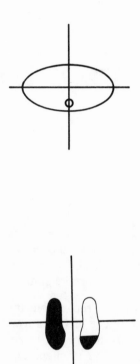

Step very slowly
to the left about
a shoulder's width;
touch only the left
toes down to the
ground.

Figure 5

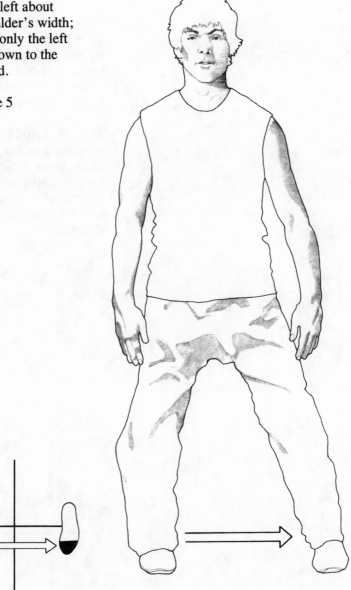

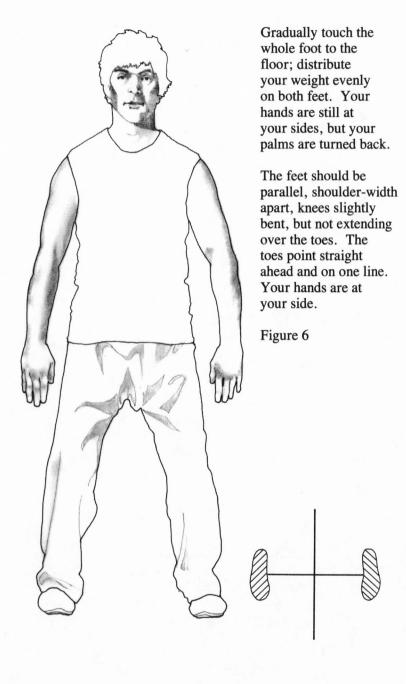

Gradually touch the
whole foot to the
floor; distribute
your weight evenly
on both feet. Your
hands are still at
your sides, but your
palms are turned back.

The feet should be
parallel, shoulder-width
apart, knees slightly
bent, but not extending
over the toes. The
toes point straight
ahead and on one line.
Your hands are at
your side.

Figure 6

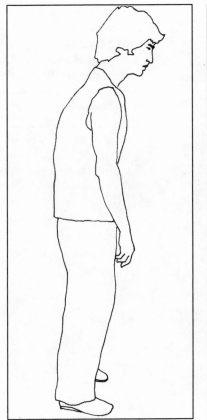 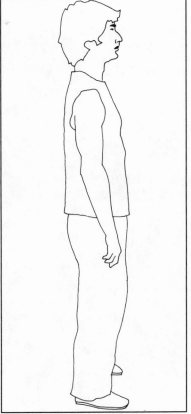

Figure 7 (side view)　　　　Figure 8 (side view)

Note the difference between Figures 7 and 8. Figure 7 is incorrect spine alignment, Figure 8 is correct alignment. This correct posture is achieved by tucking the lower part of the spine inward. You can check to see that the whole back is flat by pressing against a wall. Remember, bring the pelvis forward until the spine is perpendicular to the ground. This strengthens the flow of Chi since aligning the spine takes tension out of the whole body. Take care to keep the abdominal muscles relaxed.

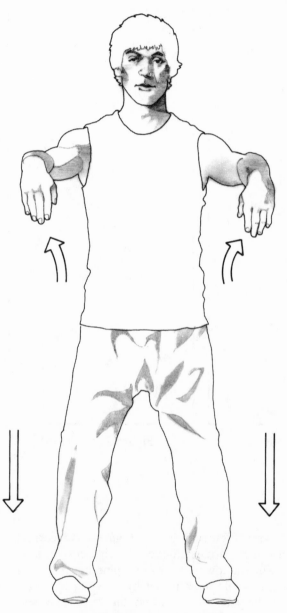

With the head
and spine straight,
sit a little,
very slowly raising
and extending the
arms with the palms
down; the wrists,
shoulders, and
elbows are relaxed.

Figure 9

As you bend the knees slightly, very slowly raise the arms to the height of your shoulders, parallel to the ground and apart one shoulder-width. Be sure to keep the shoulders and elbows relaxed.

Figure 10

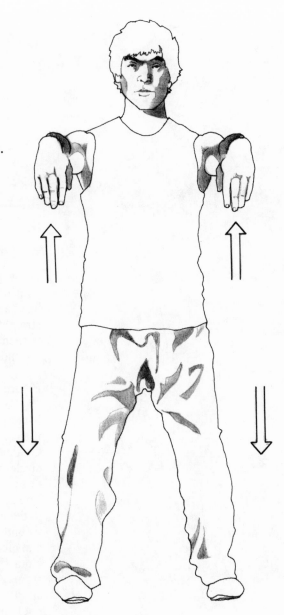

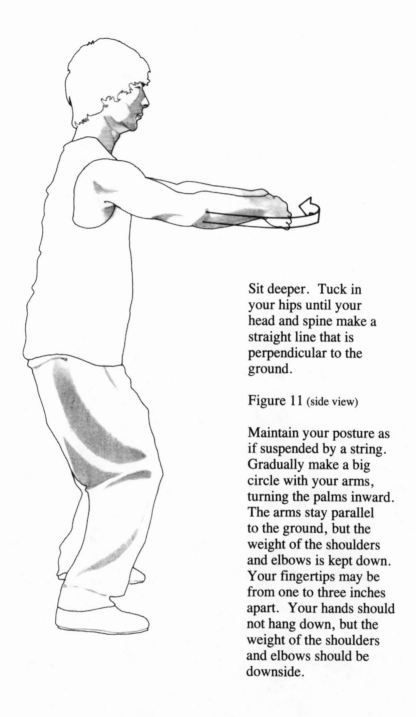

Sit deeper. Tuck in your hips until your head and spine make a straight line that is perpendicular to the ground.

Figure 11 (side view)

Maintain your posture as if suspended by a string. Gradually make a big circle with your arms, turning the palms inward. The arms stay parallel to the ground, but the weight of the shoulders and elbows is kept down. Your fingertips may be from one to three inches apart. Your hands should not hang down, but the weight of the shoulders and elbows should be downside.

After some practice you may begin to feel the Chi hold up your arms. For some experienced practitioners, the Chi force becomes so strong, they feel like their arms are lying on a table.

Figure 12

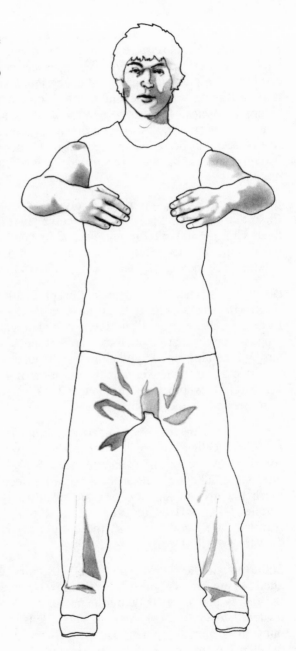

The wrists, elbows, shoulders, and the whole body are now relaxed. Hold this posture as long as you can, *without tension* or strain. A positive effect will be experienced as a warm feeling resulting in a gradual opening up of the joints and stretching of the muscles, along with a general tonification of internal organs and external muscles. Gradually increase the time spent in this posture to ten or fifteen minutes. If you create too much tension, the positive effects will be reduced. Bear in mind that this posture should be done with a calm and serene mind, relaxed body, and meditative attitude.

It is helpful to keep in mind a variety of points about this exercise. First, don't force the posture and become tense. The idea is to cultivate Chi, not to build big muscles. Carry out all steps as continuous action. Do not make stops, choppy motions, or breaks in the pattern. The movement of T'ai Chi is always fluid and continuous.

Breathing is important. Breathe deeply, slowly, and from the diaphragm. Inhale through the nose as if you were siphoning air from the outside and fill the lungs completely. This will increase lung capacity and strengthen the cardiovascular system. In particular, by breathing slowly you allow for the interaction of oxygen and carbon dioxide, increasing the oxygenation of your blood and rejuvenating the whole body. A single breath cycle may take from thirty seconds to more than a minute.

Since this posture resembles sitting on a horse it is sometimes called the Horse Riding Posture or simply The Horse. For the same reason, it is also called the Chinese Chair. Still, the root of this posture is the bubbling well at the sole of the feet. The heels lightly touch the ground and the feet are evenly aligned and precisely parallel. The knees are bent so that the lower body forms an inverted "U;" however, the knees must not be allowed to come forward over the toes.

Some practitioners argue that one must turn the toes inward to attend to the classical maxim of "the inward essence of the knees," the energy that "keeps you on the horse." For beginners this has a tendency to close the joints and create tension. Turning the feet outward is also a problem as this will make it more difficult to develop the inward essence and strength. At first, keep the feet parallel and even. Later, you may vary the posture to achieve special effects.

The major benefits of this exercise come from long-term practice. Principally, Holding the Ball benefits the digestive system. Daily practice strengthens digestion, assimilation, and elimination. After ten minutes of Holding the Ball, your whole body will heat up, from top to bottom. This internal heat helps open the joints and contributes to a gradual and general tonification of the internal organs and external muscles. The Map of T'ai Chi, Holding the Ball, opens all the joints stimulates all the meridians and cultivates the Chi.

Earth
The Receptive

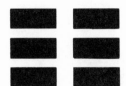

Bending
from the Waist

A cauldron with legs upturned furthers the removal of stagnancy.''
— I Ching

This exercise completes a first "movement" of the complete symphony and all three should be learned and practiced together in a single session. Don't go on to the next posture until you have developed some fluidity; practice at least one week.

Between each bending at the waist in this exercise, you sink and stand again. While you sink, inhale once and keep the spine perpendicular to the ground. When you stand, exhale, coordinating the breath and the movement. This begins a new stage of breathing, coordination of breath. Don't force coordination with the posture. If you do, it will create tension and defeat your purpose. It is said that in T'ai Chi the breath guides the movement and the mind guides the breath.

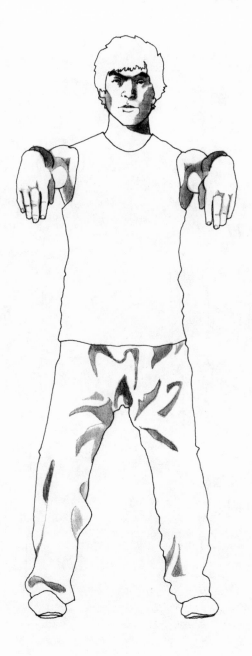

Beginning where
Holding the Ball
left off, extend
the arms gradually,
palms down.

Figure 13

The wrists are relaxed. Simultaneously and gradually stand straight and let the hands float down to the sides of the body as though you were swimming in air, but keep your weight underside!

Figure 14

The knees are straight but not locked; the coccyx and back are straight.

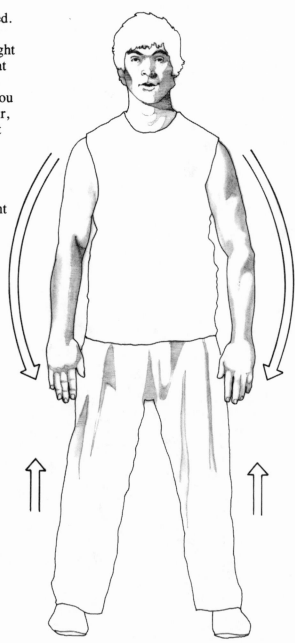

The arms and whole body are relaxed and alive. Keep the back straight and start bending from the waist, extending the head forward.

Figure 15

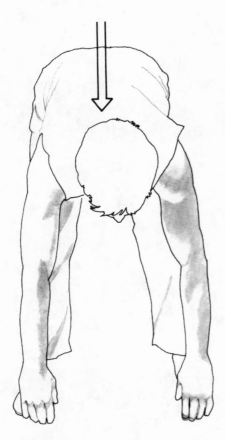

Emphasize stretching the major muscle groups behind the legs and lower back. You are working toward a spring-like flexibility in the whole of the spine.

Remember to keep the feet parallel so that when you bend from the waist, you can also stretch the connective tissue in the ankles, knees, and hips. Keep your breathing diaphragmatic, natural. Exhale and inhale when you need to.

Look back between the legs in a continual motion. The knees are kept straight but not locked. Stop when you obtain the maximum stretch in the legs.

Figure 16

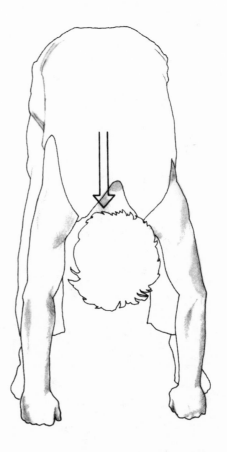

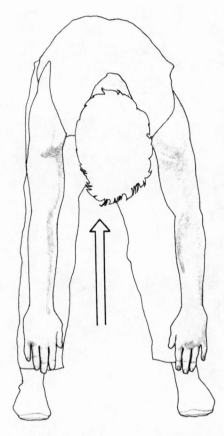

Avoid tensing. The movement is slow and even. Pause a second or two looking back between the legs.

Then, gradually start coming up, continuing to look back. The knees are still straight; but relax the back so you get a "rolling action" in the spine. This is one of the few times when we bend the spine. Yet the head, neck, and spine have a bow-like alignment.

Figure 17

Come up to a
straight, relaxed
position.

Figure 18

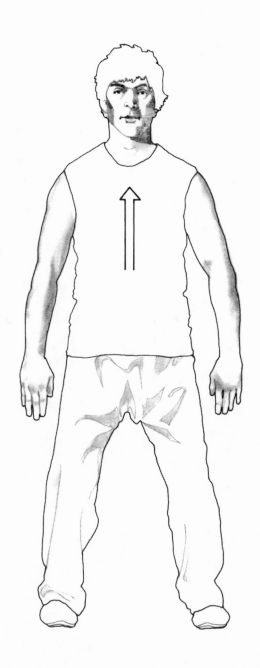

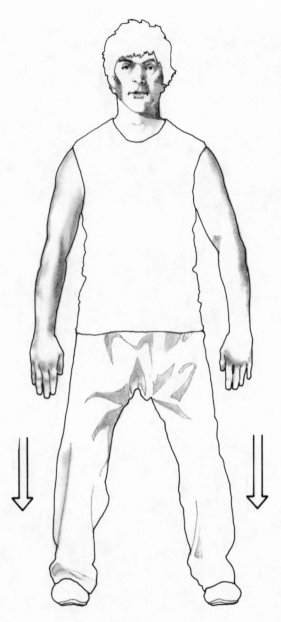

With the head and spine straight, sit slowly bending the knees. Take care that the knees do not extend over the toes and that your head and spine are ''suspended from a string.'' Inhale.

Figure 19

Exhaling, stand
again slowly and
relax with the
back straight.

Figure 20

Then, bend from the
waist as at the
beginning of this
movement and repeat
a second time
(Figure 14 to 20).
Then, bend a third
time (Figure 14 to 18).

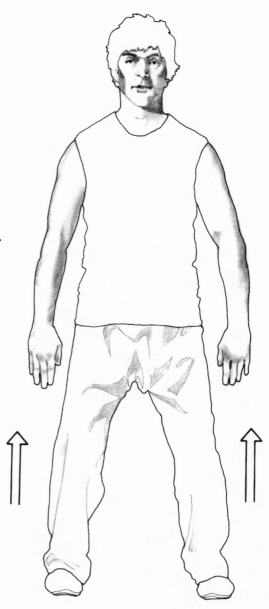

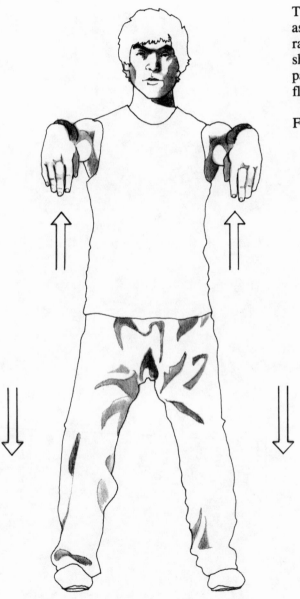

The third time,
as you sit straight,
raise the arms to
shoulder height,
parallel to the
floor.

Figure 21

Now sit deeper,
returning to the
Map of T'ai Chi.

Figure 22

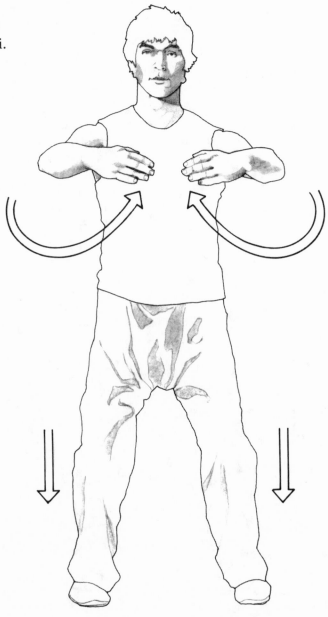

Except for the mentioned pauses, the movements should be slow, smooth, and continuous. Do three repetitions, slowly, taking two to five minutes. These three preceding forms, Preparation, Holding the Ball, and Bending from the Waist, should be learned in one sitting. Do not attempt the next movement for at least one week, but practice these three daily. Done slowly, these three movements may take seven to twenty minutes depending on rhythm and how long we "hold the ball."

The essential benefits of Bending from the Waist are a general and systemic elasticity and resiliency in the muscles. The spine too is flexed and strengthened. Bending forward, as in this exercise, is a feature of a number of Oriental exercises that tonify the liver, bladder, and gallbladder. Coming up from the sitting posture benefits the kidneys, spleen, and stomach. All the meridians in the legs are tonified and stimulated.

Since your body will be changing, stretching, and lengthening ligaments and muscles and opening joints, there may be some soreness. If you have much pain during practice, try to relax more. Go only as far as you can without tension. T'ai Chi emphasizes complete relaxation, never tension. In order to gain full benefit, it is important to learn to relax through the tension and tightness that you may experience in the beginning. If you have time, do more repetitions, but never less than three.

Fire
The Clinging

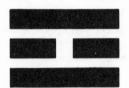

Riding A
T'ai Chi Horse

"The Yielding receives the honored place in the great middle;
the upper and the lower correspond with it."
— *I Ching*

Y ou may move directly into Riding a T'ai Chi Horse after you have begun to feel and experience coherence in the first three postures. You should be sitting deeper in Holding the Ball. Showing some stamina, up to ten minutes of Holding the Ball should feel good, not strained. You should be making all three movements a continuous flow. This movement, Riding a T'ai Chi Horse, consists of T'ai Chi leg raises. You must be at ease with the previous postures or the attempt to learn this exercise will result in a lot of ineffective motion. Do the movements slowly, with relaxation and Chi extension.

Coordinating mind and body is a recurring theme in T'ai Chi. This is difficult, sometimes it's hard enough just to coordinate your arms and legs. Remember Tohei's principle of keeping one point, the Tan Tien center. It is imperative that you keep the head and spine aligned and as close to perpendicular to the ground as is possible. This is where having kept your head "suspended from a string" in Preparation pays off.

The leg that carries the weight is called the Yang leg; conversely the "light" leg is Yin. In T'ai Chi we are not simply exercising the Yang leg, but also the non-weighted or Yin leg. Paradoxically, the non-weighted, Yin leg may be considered as Yang in the sense that it is in greater motion. The Yang leg is exercised too, in that the muscles and ligaments are stretched. This is why it is important not to extend the knee over the toes, over-reaching or over-stretching both the leg and your balance.

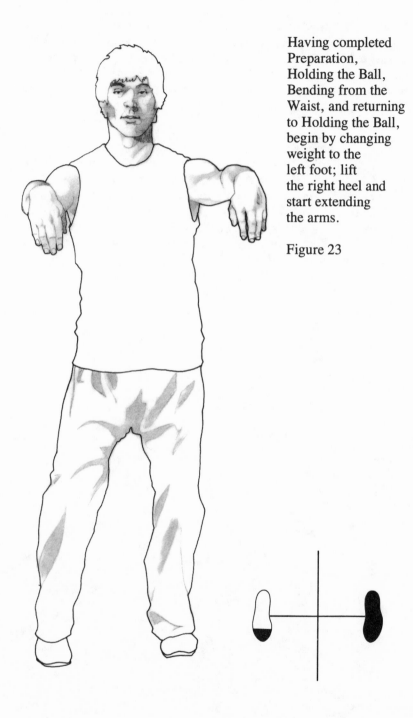

Having completed
Preparation,
Holding the Ball,
Bending from the
Waist, and returning
to Holding the Ball,
begin by changing
weight to the
left foot; lift
the right heel and
start extending
the arms.

Figure 23

Take a half-step inward with the right foot while extending the arms out, palms down. The wrists, elbows, and shoulders are relaxed, the arms are shoulder-width apart and parallel to the ground.

Figure 24

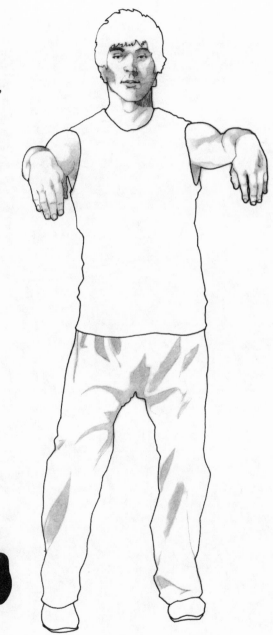

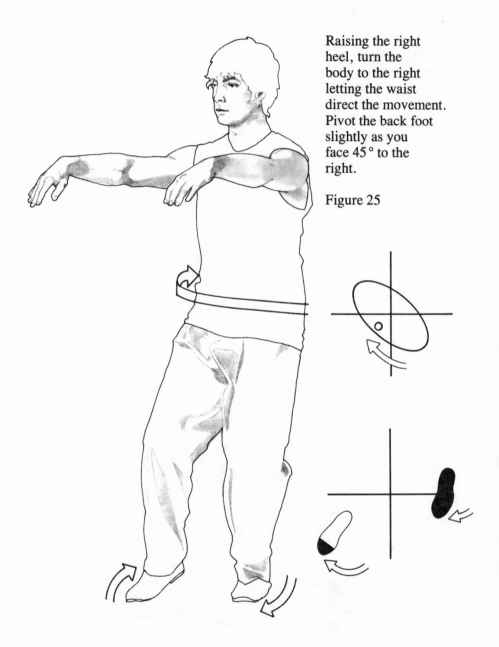

Raising the right heel, turn the body to the right letting the waist direct the movement. Pivot the back foot slightly as you face 45° to the right.

Figure 25

Gradually lower your arms to the sides of the body, keeping the palms down; sit deeper on the left leg.

Figure 26

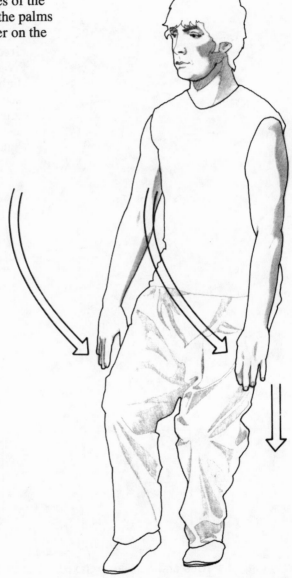

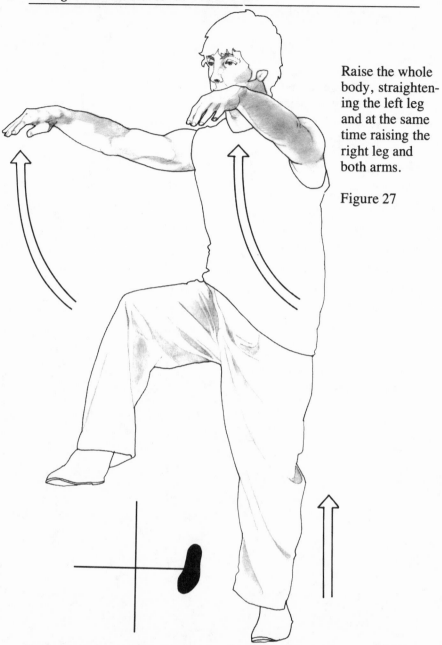

Raise the whole body, straightening the left leg and at the same time raising the right leg and both arms.

Figure 27

Here, both the arms and legs are relaxed. The right knee is bent and the right leg extends outward slightly while the left knee is just slightly bent. The shoulders, wrists, and elbows are relaxed. The arms are shoulder-width apart, at eye level; the palms are down.

When you reach the high point, slowly lower the body by bending the left leg and at the same time bring the arms down gradually along with the right leg.

The right leg comes slightly in. The right heel is slightly raised and the left leg carries almost all the weight.

Figure 28

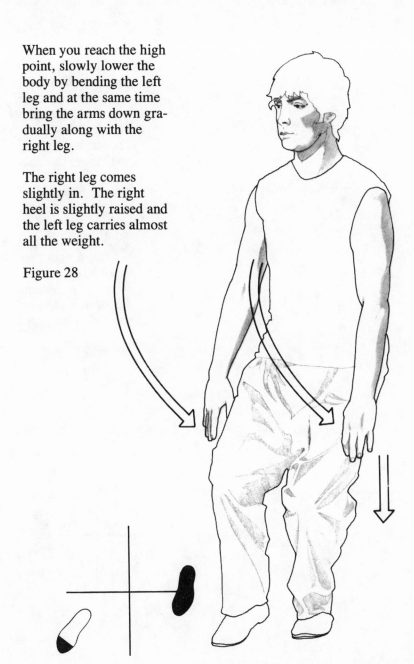

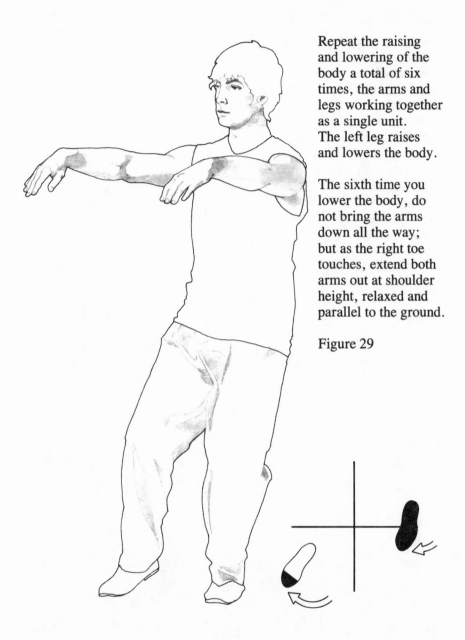

Repeat the raising and lowering of the body a total of six times, the arms and legs working together as a single unit. The left leg raises and lowers the body.

The sixth time you lower the body, do not bring the arms down all the way; but as the right toe touches, extend both arms out at shoulder height, relaxed and parallel to the ground.

Figure 29

While keeping the weight on the left leg, turn from the waist 90° to the left. Pivot 45° to the left on the right toe, then shift the weight to the right foot. The left foot pivots 45° to the left as the weight shifts to the right foot. Your body will now face left at 45°.

Figure 30

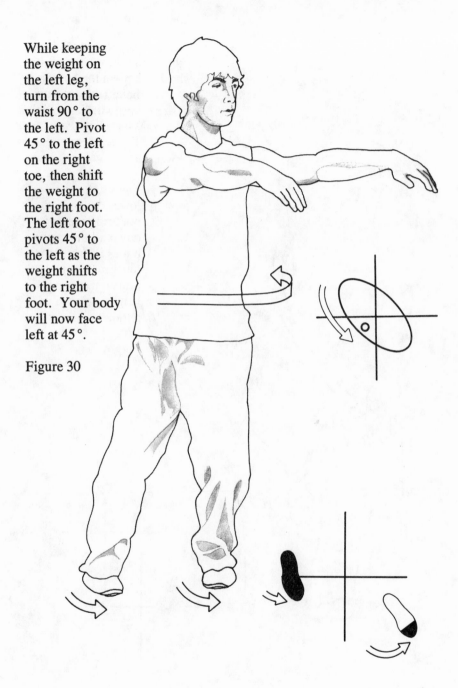

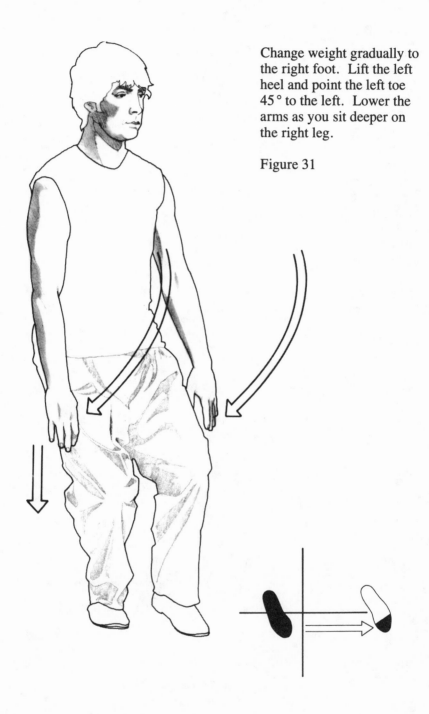

Change weight gradually to the right foot. Lift the left heel and point the left toe 45° to the left. Lower the arms as you sit deeper on the right leg.

Figure 31

Raise and lower
yourself on the
right leg, just
as you did on
the left leg, a
total of six times.

Figure 32

Remember to
keep your back
straight and
move the arms
and leg as a
single unit.

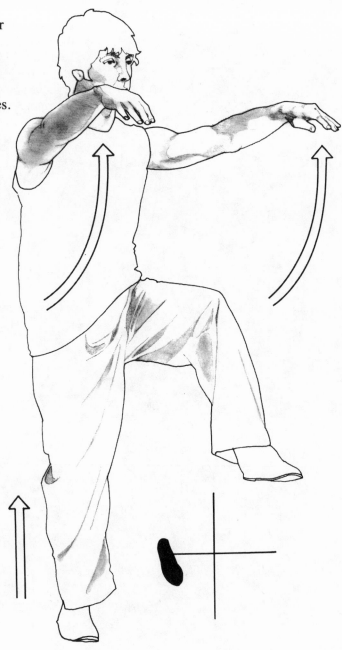

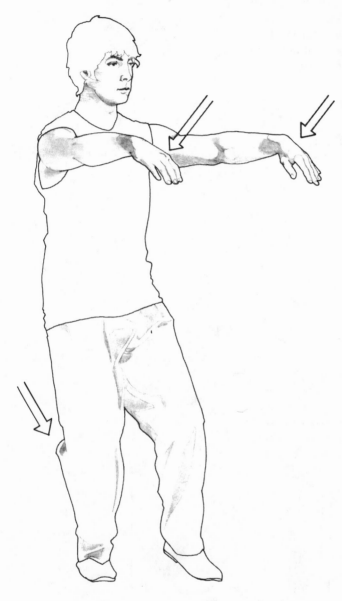

The sixth time, as the left toe touches the ground, the arms come down just a little and extend, relaxed, shoulder-width apart.

Figure 33

Now the waist directs the body
to the right. The weight is on
the right leg and your left foot
turns 45° to the right until your
left toe points forward.

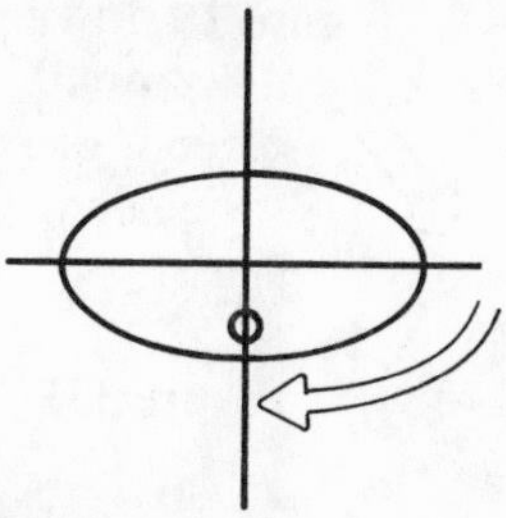

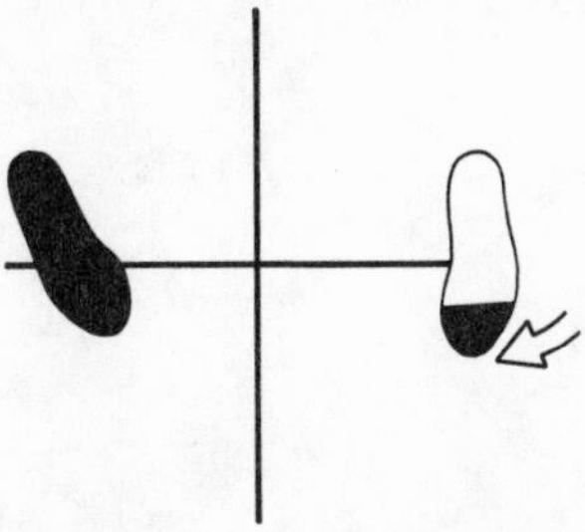

Change your weight to the
left foot, turn your right
foot forward on the right heel.
Your body now faces forward
with the weight evenly distributed on both legs. Sink lower,
keeping the back straight.

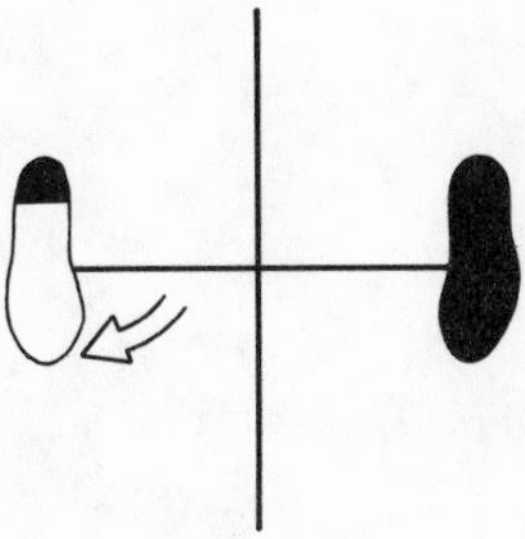

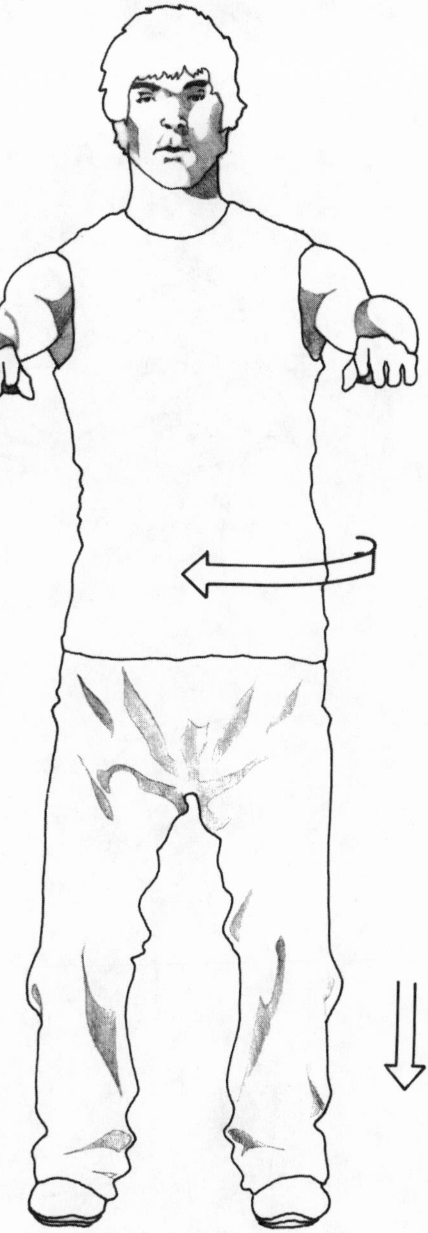

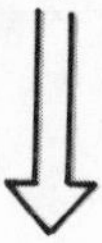

Figure 34

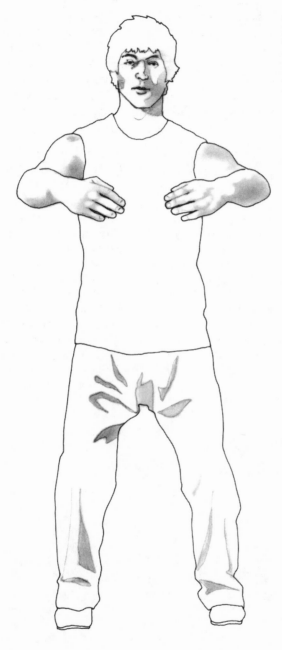

Return to the
Map of T'ai Chi
(Holding the Ball).

Figure 35

Keeping your balance here is very difficult. If you keep your back straight, keep your center of gravity over the rooted leg, maintain relaxation, and avoid forcing the movement, you will attain facility with time. It is also important to keep the mind calm. Do not go on to the next movement until this one can be done smoothly, continuously, and slowly for about two minutes on each leg. Practice this in conjunction with the preceding three forms for about one week. Then proceed to the next movement.

With the circular dynamics of this movement, you will be opening the joints and the pull will greatly strengthen your legs. The Yin leg is aligned, and relaxed to the deepest muscles. The Kidney Meridians on both legs are stimulated, particularly by keeping your weight at the bubbling well. The exercise also greatly strengthens the heart and is particularly useful for people with weak cardiovascular systems.

It's important to note that T'ai Chi is a metabolic regulator. On one hand, working the body strengthens the natural rhythms and each internal system stimulates the next. On the other hand, the flow of stimulation allows any extremes to come into a more harmonious balance. For example, a very nervous and excitable person can work on relaxation and keeping weight downside. A weak person who lacks energy can concentrate on Chi extension.

Water
The Abysmal

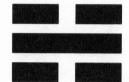

Springy Step

"Drinking from the clear cold spring
depends upon its central and correct position."
— *I Ching*

Many Chinese poetic names come from nature. For example, Sweep Lotus with Foot, Push the Mountain into the Sea, Stork Spreads Wings and Climb Mountain on Tigers Back. We too come from nature and in T'ai Chi we learn from nature, as this movement is sometimes referred to as the Tiger Walk.

For me, doing T'ai Chi is like taking a walk along a mountain path where every new step and turn produces a beautiful panorama. A tiger steps lightly. They are nimble, sure-footed, and secure. Elephants are also sure-footed and secure, but without the springing vitality of a tiger. I caution you that in T'ai Chi it is more beneficial to step like a cat than to walk like an elephant. To add image to image, the tiger walks like the swift current of a long river. Thus, the T'ai Chi adage that T'ai Chi is "in movement like the long flowing river and in stillness like the tall mountain."

This is the first posture where you will be taking full steps; make sure you are rooted and secure. Follow principles not just at the beginning and end of your steps, but at all the infinite number of points in between. Again, be sure that the previous four movements can be done relaxed, with principle, with fluidity, and Chi extension before your undertake the Springy Step.

From the end of
the last posture,
extend your arms
out in front of
you, hands down.

Figure 36

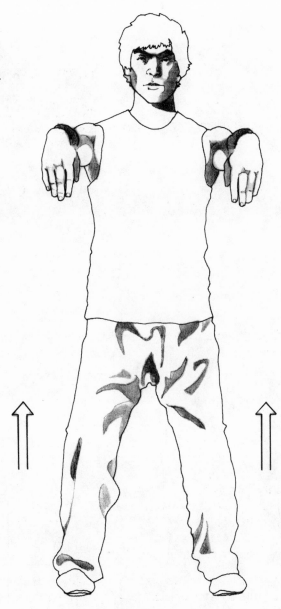

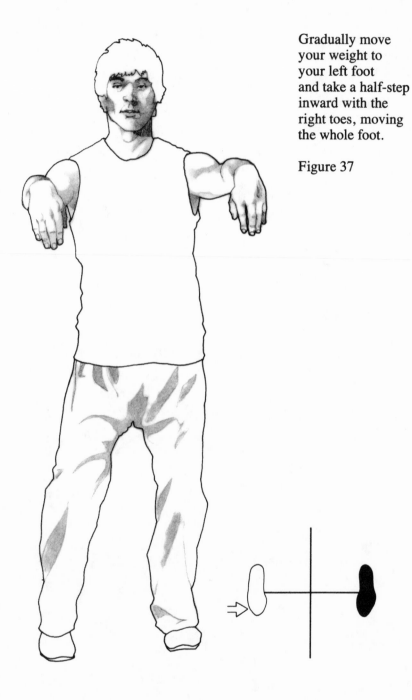

Gradually move
your weight to
your left foot
and take a half-step
inward with the
right toes, moving
the whole foot.

Figure 37

Turn your body at the waist 90° to the right. At the same time, pivot your left foot 45° to the right, while shifting the position on your right foot from toe to heel (turn 90° to the right).

Figure 38

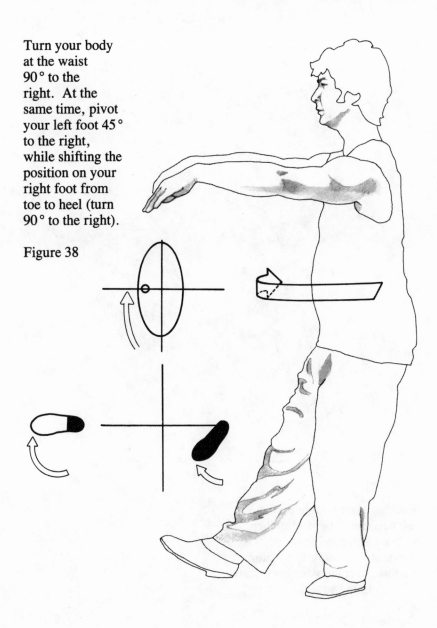

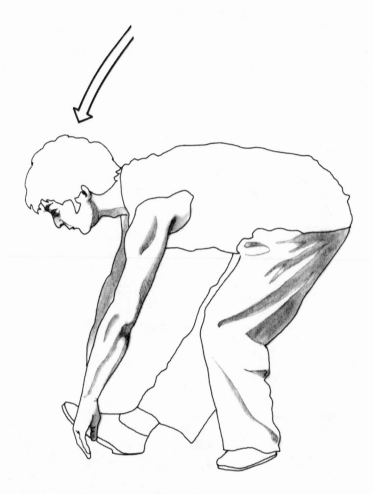

Keeping your weight on the left
leg which will be slightly bent,
sit back and bend forward. Go
down as far as you can without
tension, keeping your back and
your right leg straight.

Figure 39

Sit back into the hip. Put as little weight as possible on the front foot so as to open the hip joints. Keep the leg in front of you stretched and naturally straight.

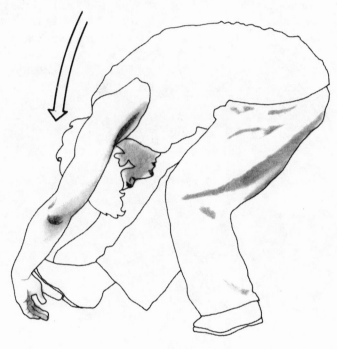

Figure 40

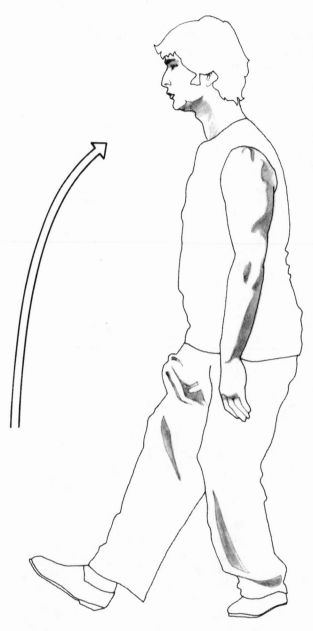

Rise back up, keeping your left leg bent and your right leg straight. Roll the spine as you come up, just as you did in Touching the Earth.

Figure 41

Turn your right foot to the right 45°. Allow your waist to direct the movement of the foot (keep your left leg bent).

Figure 42

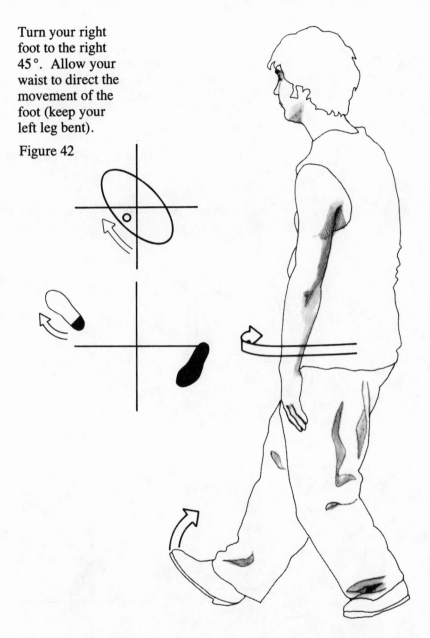

When moving with the ''Springy Step'' keep your hands next to the body and the weight going down. Don't use your arms for counter-balance. Learn to be not only balanced but rooted and centered.

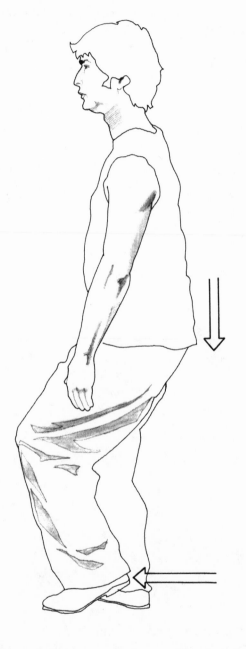

Change weight to
your right foot.
Lift your left heel
and step up.

Sit a little on the
right leg by bending
your right knee.

Figure 43

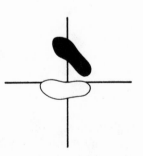

Stand straight on your right leg; swing your left foot forward slightly, toes pointing straight ahead.   Figure 44

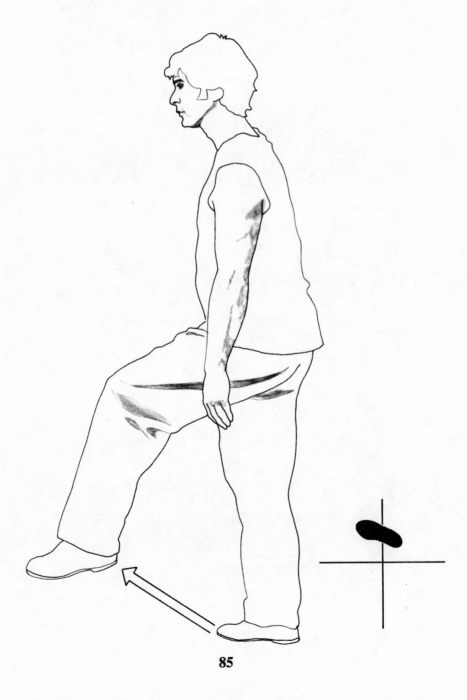

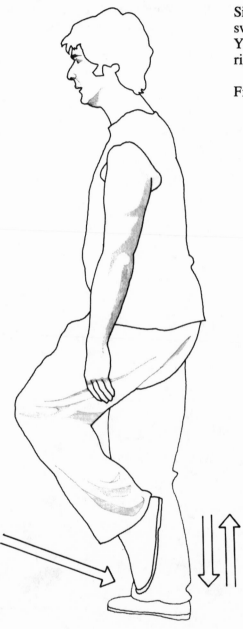

Sink on the right leg and swing your left foot back. Your left toe is next to your right leg.

Figure 45

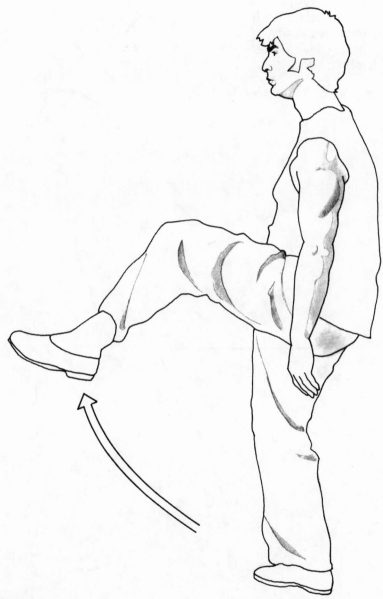

Figure 46

Sink on your right leg; as you stand, swing your left foot outward as straight and as high as you can without tensing.

Sinking slightly on your
right leg, let the left leg
come down slowly,
touching down on the
left heel.

Figure 47

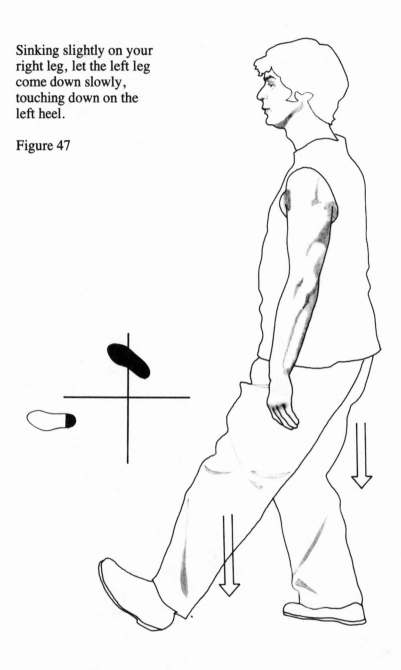

As before, bend forward, but keep your weight on the right leg. Come up as before, rolling the spine.

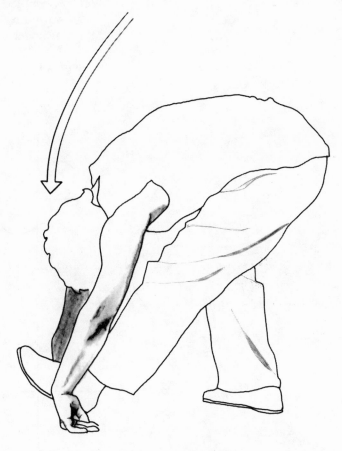

Figure 48

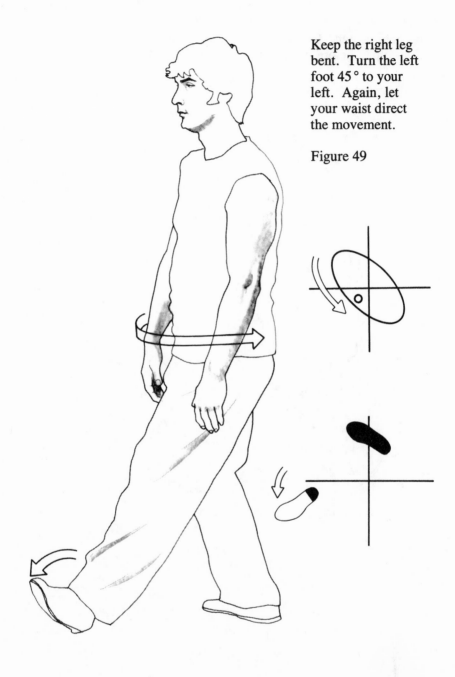

Keep the right leg bent. Turn the left foot 45° to your left. Again, let your waist direct the movement.

Figure 49

Move forward,
bringing your
left foot down,
and change your
weight to the
left foot.

Figure 50

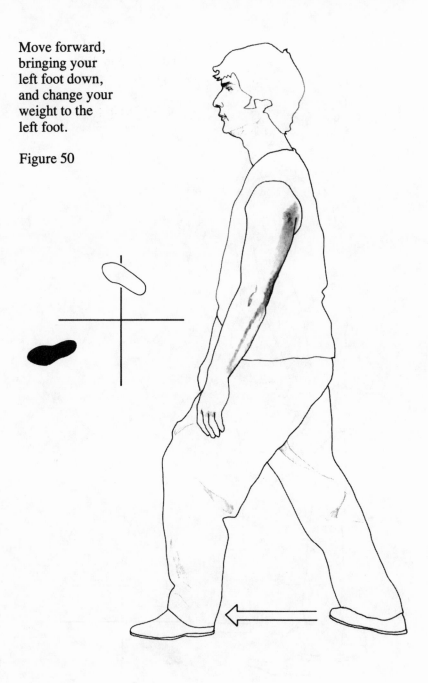

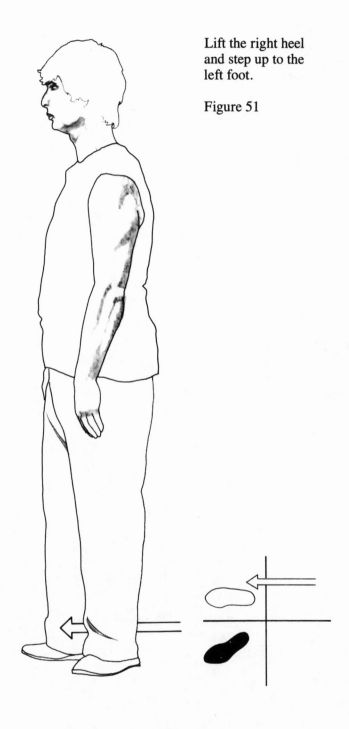

Lift the right heel
and step up to the
left foot.

Figure 51

Repeat this sitting and
swinging procedure with
your weight on your left
leg (Figure 43 to 47,
with weight on the left
foot).

Figure 52

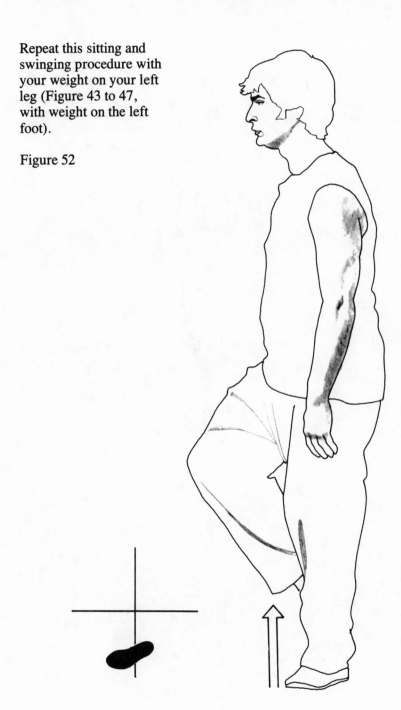

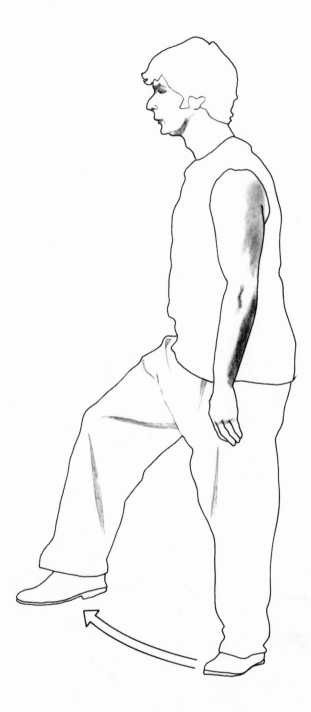

Don't kick the leg out; let it swing freely and keep your weight on the bubbling well.

Figure 53

As before, sink
slightly, this time
with your weight
on your left leg,
touching down on
the right heel.

Figure 54

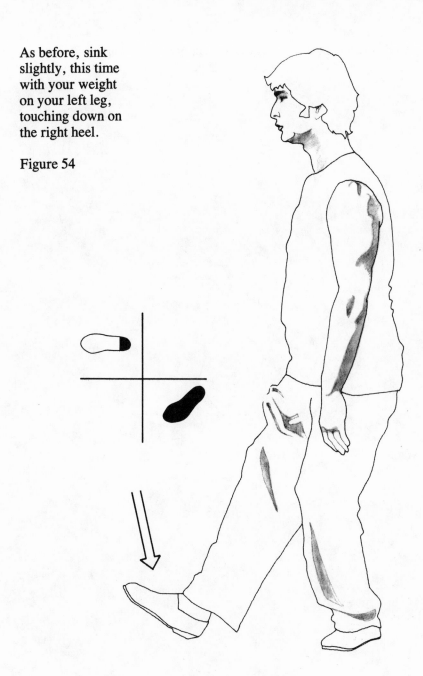

Again bend forward, with your weight on your left leg.

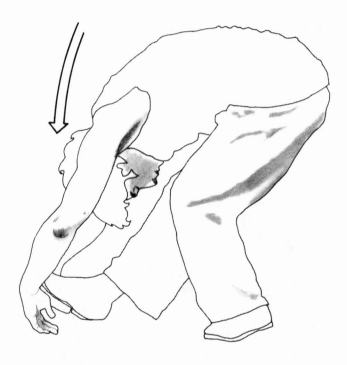

Figure 55

As before, roll the spine as you come up, returning to the upright position, while keeping the left leg bent.

Figure 56

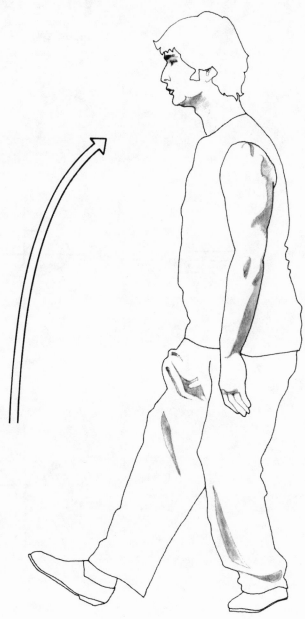

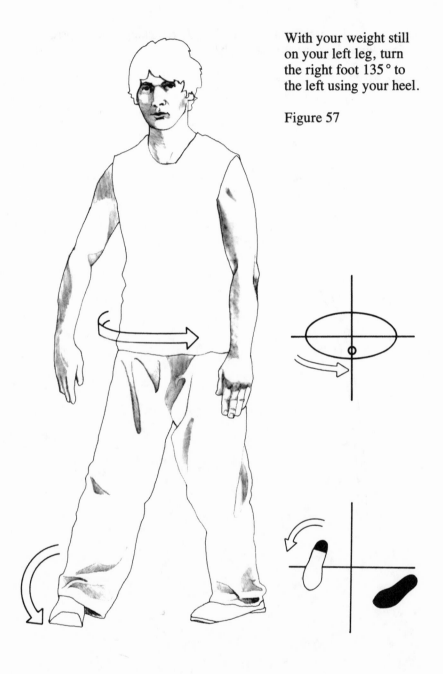

With your weight still on your left leg, turn the right foot 135° to the left using your heel.

Figure 57

As you change weight to
the right foot, lift the left
heel and stand straight
on the right leg, drawing
back your left foot to be
even with your right
foot. You are now fac-
ing 180° in the opposite
direction.

Figure 58

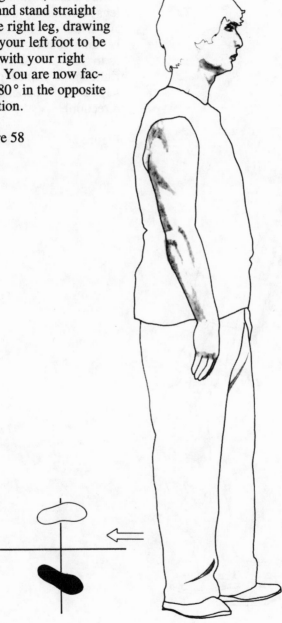

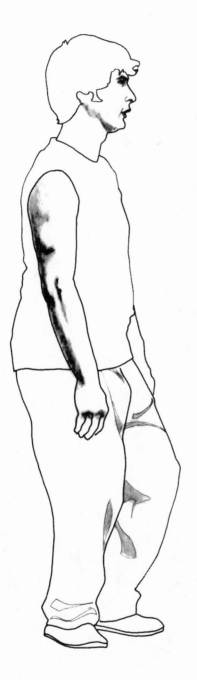

Repeat the exercise from bending and swinging your legs while facing the opposite direction. Start with bending your right knee so as to ''sit'' a little on your right leg (as from Figure 43, but in the opposite direction).

Figure 59

As you do this, concentrate on keeping your breathing soft and relaxed and your spine perpendicular.

Figure 60

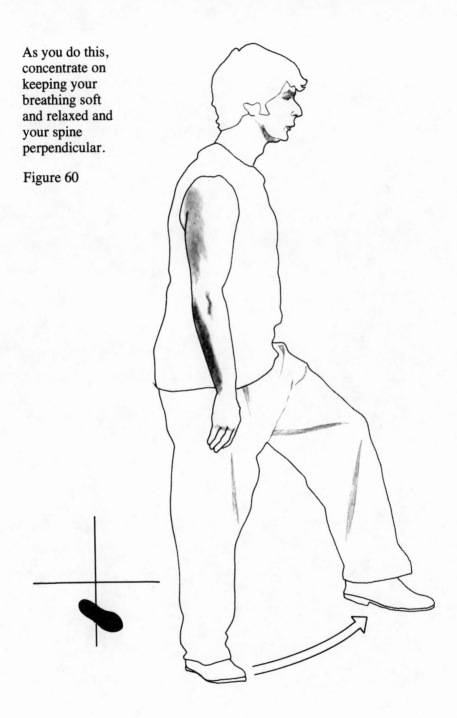

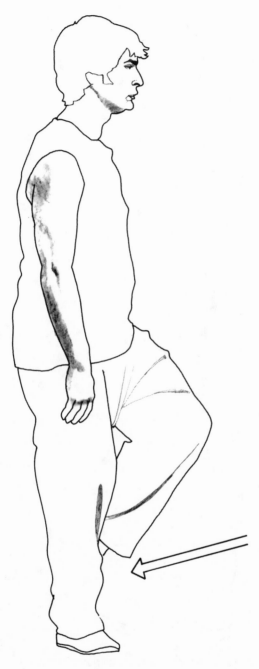

Remember that the
leg swings freely.

Figure 61

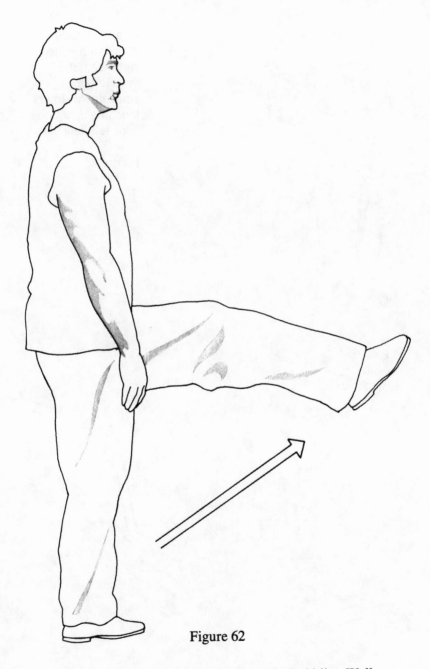

Figure 62

Remember to keep your weight on the Bubbling Well.

103

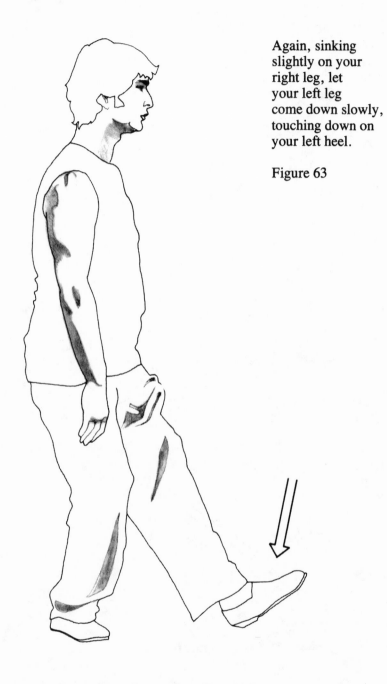

Again, sinking
slightly on your
right leg, let
your left leg
come down slowly,
touching down on
your left heel.

Figure 63

Again bend forward,
with your weight on
your right leg.

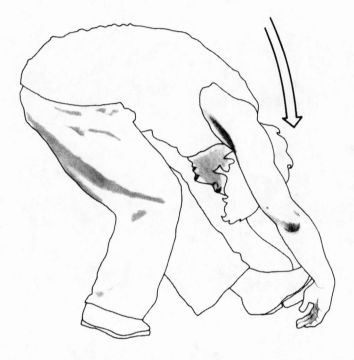

Figure 64

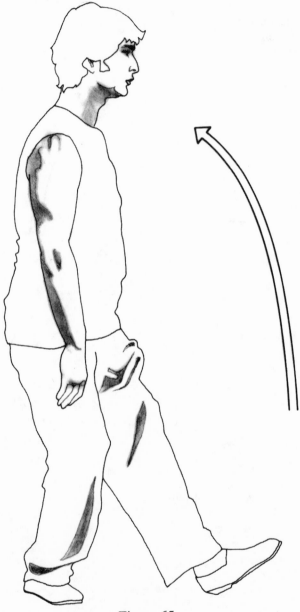

Figure 65

As before, roll the spine as you come up, returning to the upright position, while keeping the right leg bent.

Keep your right
leg bent. Turn
you left leg 45°
to the left, using
your waist to direct
the movement.

Figure 66

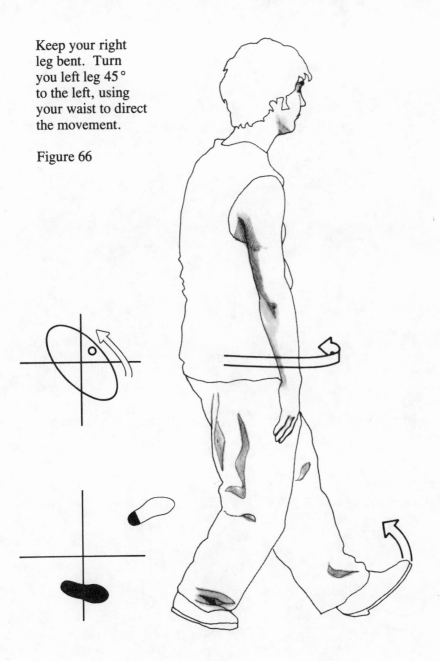

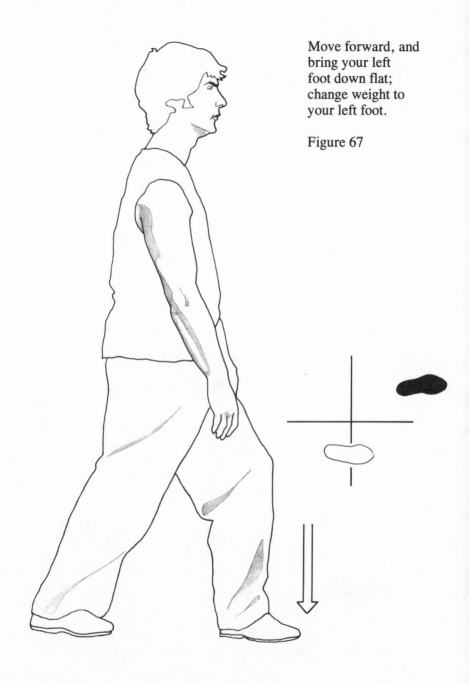

Move forward, and
bring your left
foot down flat;
change weight to
your left foot.

Figure 67

Lift the right heel and
step up. The right foot is
weightless, positioned
slightly in advance of the
left foot.

Figure 68

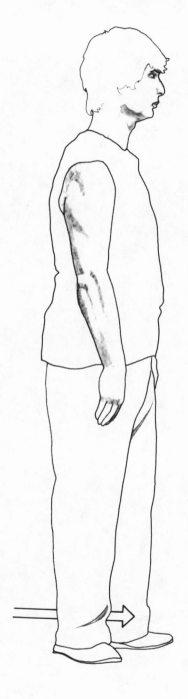

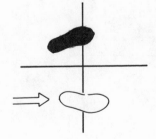

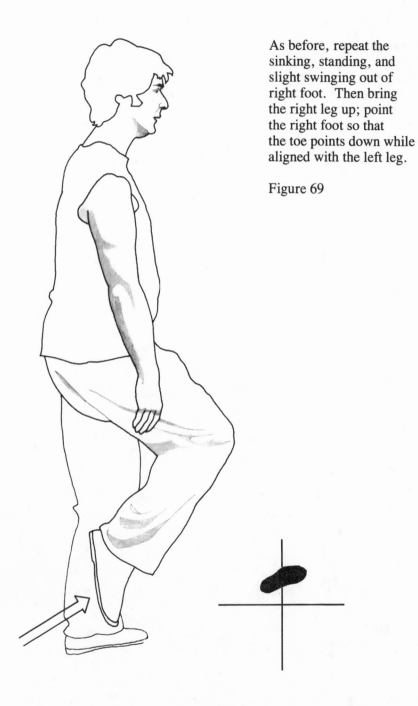

As before, repeat the sinking, standing, and slight swinging out of right foot. Then bring the right leg up; point the right foot so that the toe points down while aligned with the left leg.

Figure 69

Now swing it out freely, keeping your weight centered on the Bubbling Well.

Figure 70

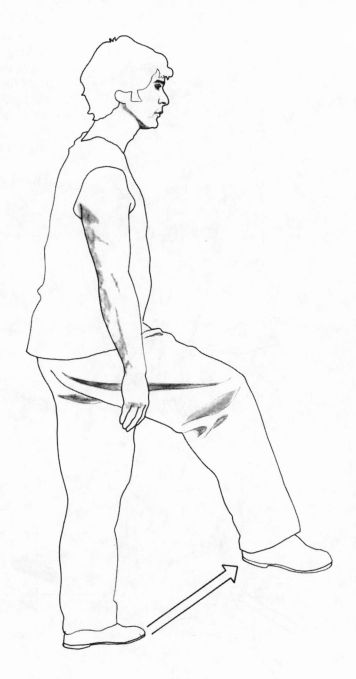

Bring your right heel
down, sinking a little
at the knee.

Figure 71

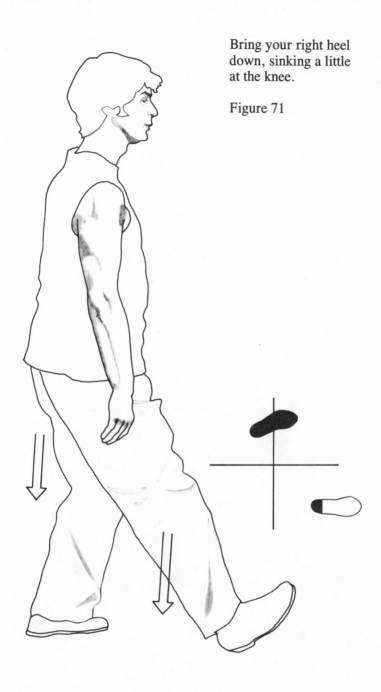

Bend forward, keeping your weight on your left leg. Again, roll the spine as you come to an upright position.

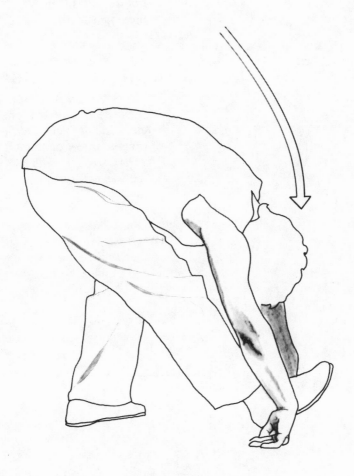

Figure 72

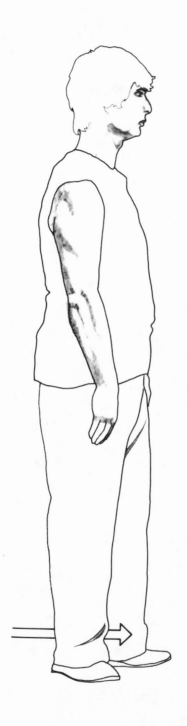

Turn the right foot
out and step up as
before, still facing
the opposite direction.

Figure 73

Repeat swinging the leg
and bending a final time.
Make sure your steps are
clear and defined. Don't
drag your feet or stumble
as you step up. The path of
the step describes an
inward arc.

Don't look down at your
feet while you step. Both
feet will still be there at the
end of the exercise.

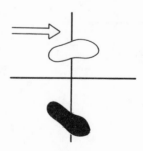

Turn the left foot
forward 90°
using the heel.

Figure 74

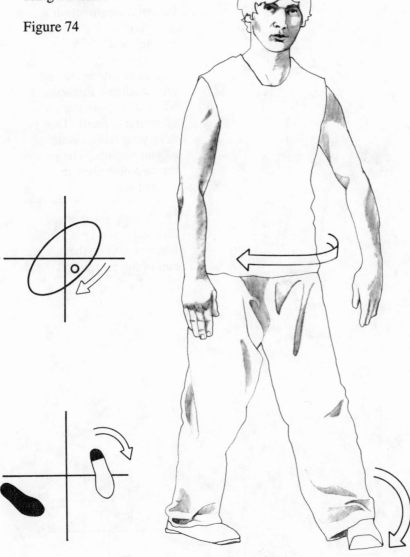

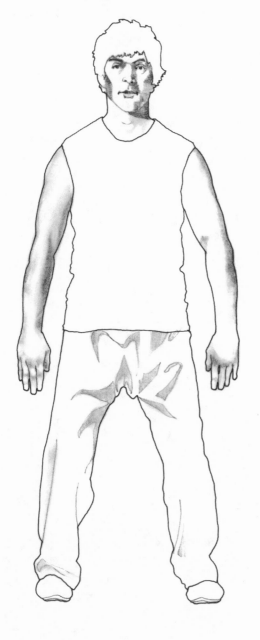

Change weight to
your left leg.
Lift your right
toe; turn your
right foot on
the heel 45°
forward. Center
your weight on
both feet and sink.

Figure 75

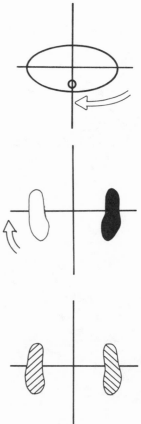

Bring your arms up,
keeping your fingertips
slightly down and
curved naturally to
the ground. Sink a
little more at the
knees.

Figure 76

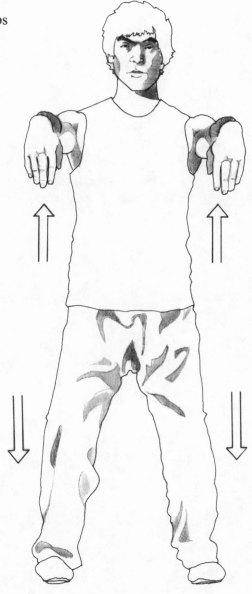

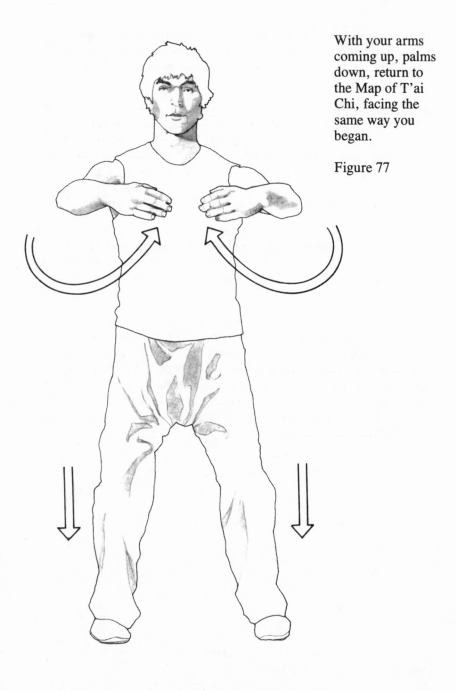

With your arms coming up, palms down, return to the Map of T'ai Chi, facing the same way you began.

Figure 77

This movement is called the Springy Step because it develops springiness in the legs. In particular, this movement opens up the ankle joints and hip, complementing the previous posture, Riding a T'ai Chi Horse.

In summation, there are three bending movements to the right and only two springy steps, and three bending movements and springy steps to the left. Again all this should be done smoothly, slowly, and continuously. The time taken should be from three to eight minutes. Be sure to avoid "double weighting" in the steps and to allow at least one week combined practice of this exercise with the previous four movements before attempting the next sequence.

By now, depending on how long you Hold the Ball and how slowly you do the movements, these first five movements may take from fifteen to thirty minutes. The last three movements are not so lengthy but the entire basic exercises may take between twenty and fifty minutes.

The more time you spend learning basics, the easier you will find attaining the next level of development. Without time it is difficult to do any lasting good. Many schools of T'ai Chi use the Springy Step as an auxilliary to their formal movements. As it is presented here it is not auxilliary but indeed fundamental. It serves to teach the fundamental ideas and dynamics of movement, develop the body, and develop the Chi. Without these basics more sophisticated T'ai Chi forms have no purpose.

Lake
The Joyous

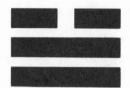

Carry Tiger Back to the Mountain

"Heaven moves steadily.
So should man exercise hmself regularly."
— *I Ching*

People have done some strange things to achieve enlightenment and happiness. We know that during the Byzantine Empire certain of the formal Christian elite had themselves neutered in order to acquire the alchemical element of immortality. In parts of India, some acetics cut off fingers or toes as a sacrifice to attain heaven. Indeed, the *I Ching* tells us "deliver yourself from your big toe."

There is certainly a possibility that some measure of enlightenment may come from cutting something off. Certainly, having done so, your first thought might be "I wish I hadn't done that." It is indeed a great revelation that you shouldn't have neutered yourself or hacked off an appendage. But the adage relating to nature is always, "at what cost?"

Striving and competition is not in the vocabulary of T'ai Chi. By striving and competition I do not mean that work which is designed to better ourselves, but rather the idea of putting others down to give us a relative feeling of well being. Many practitioners of martial arts study to improve their combative and self-defense skills. Very often during training we may take the worst beating of our

120

life. This is a dear price to pay since our original intent was to avoid taking a thrashing. Often the injuries we sustain may ruin our health and even prevent us from defending ourselves adequately. Many olympic weight-lifters sustain injuries to their joints that weaken instead of strengthen. Many marathon runners develop internal injuries that reduce their overall health. Again, the cost is too great. Trophies, medals, fame, or money cannot insure health and happiness. Realistically, sports and competition of this type prove very little. As these athletes become older their bodies wear out; at the intense competitive level this takes but a few years. Thirty-five years old becomes very old and tired.

A six-pound house cat fighting for its life can deliver great damage to the best of pugilists. A woman with her child pinned under a car could lift much more weight than the olympic medalist. An untrained individual running for their life may cover a great distance out of need, so when we train our minds and bodies we must always consider our intent and not do things simply to placate our egos or benefit at another's expense. Cultivating the Chi knows no limitation. Having faith in yourself you may rise to the occasion.

Tsao Li Ming use to follow the idea of "investing in loss." Some day to keep the body perpendicular to the ground you may not be able to sit as deeply. On another day to sit deeper you may incline your head and spine slightly. When we invest in loss, we may find a better approach. When we invest in loss, we learn humility; investing in loss may avoid costly errors. As one may not resist and yet not surrender one can retreat to a more favorable position without defeat. Softness itself is an investment in loss; we give up our physical strength and realize a strength of the spirit.

Remember, keep the body soft or it is not T'ai Chi. Keep your breath complete, relaxed and abdominal. Make your exhalations well-defined and make sure each is complete. If you can begin a movement with an inhalation, it is good, but more importantly, keep your breath relaxed.

In this posture it is important to watch your weight distribution. Keep your weight on the bubbling well; it will be easy to let your weight slip back to the heel. Then, like a tired shortstop whose energy is exhausted, you will lose your balance and flexibility. The image of this movement is walking to the shore of a lake. As you sit down near the shore you cup your hands and gather the water. As you stand, you let the water return to the sea. We are indeed not only swimming in an ocean of air, but also a sea of Chi.

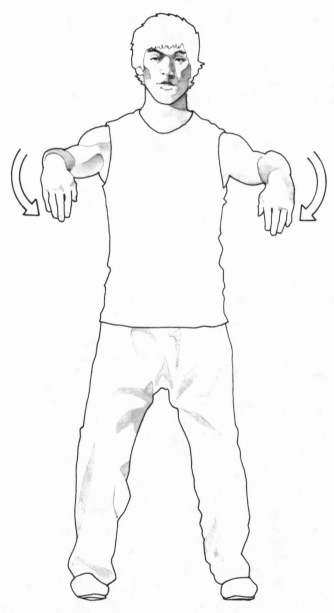

Continuing from the last posture, stand slightly, extending the arms and turning your hands downward.

Figure 78

Continue standing and extend your arms upward over your head. Your elbows are slightly bent; your finger tips extend upward.

Figure 79

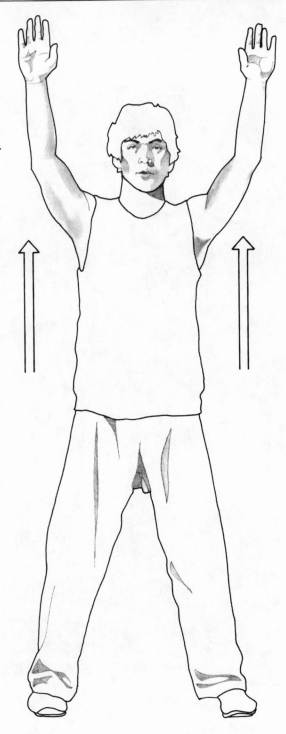

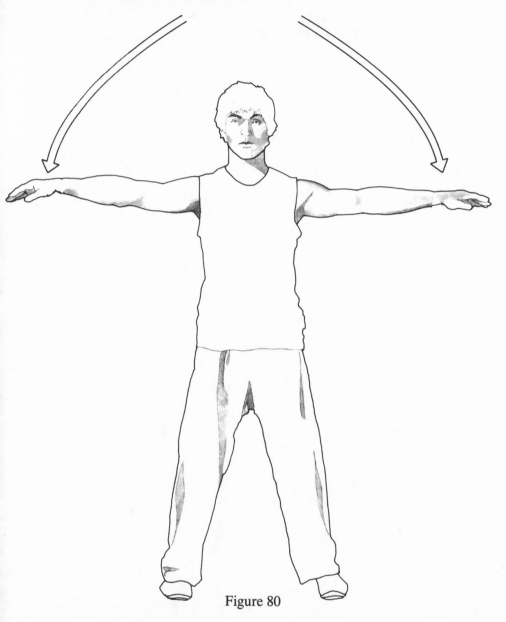

Figure 80

Carefully and slowly, bring the arms down in a big arc until they are parallel with the ground. From the corner of your right eye, watch your right hand; from the corner of your left eye, watch your left hand.

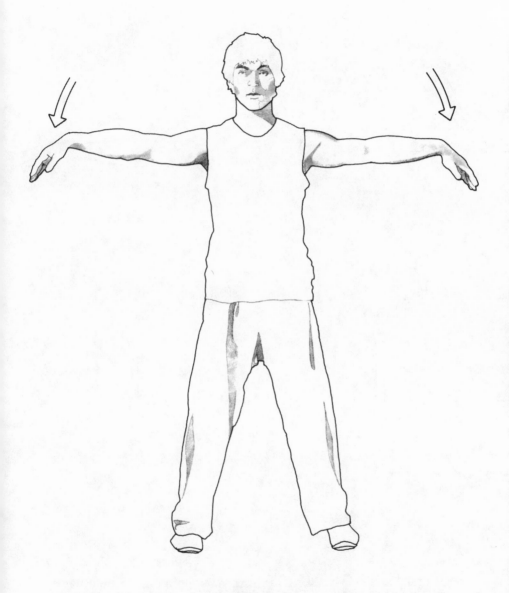

Figure 81

Look forward and relax the wrists.

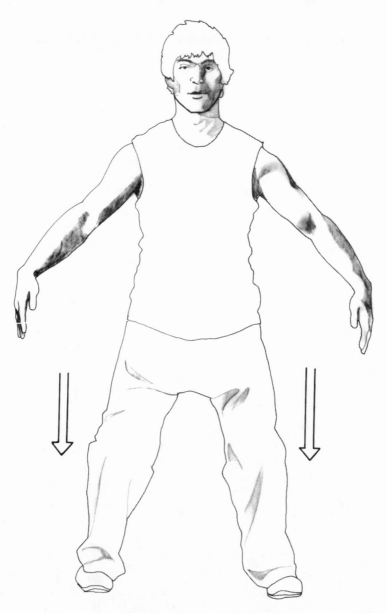

Bending your knees, sit back, keeping your head and spine straight.
Begin to lower your arms, still in a wide arc, toward your knees.

Figure 82

Arc your arms downward, brushing your knees. Make sure your knees do not extend forward beyond the toes.

Figure 83

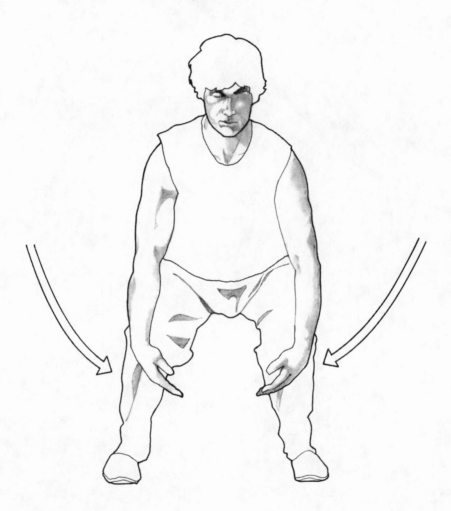

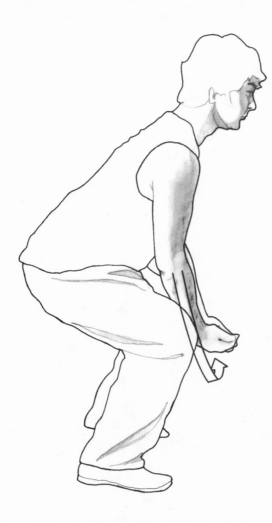

Bring your hands together. Cupping your right hand over your left hand, exhale completely.

Figure 84
(side view)

Rise slowly, keeping
your back straight.
Extend your arms in
front of you.

Figure 85

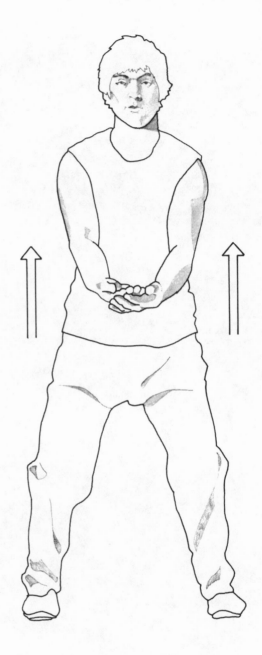

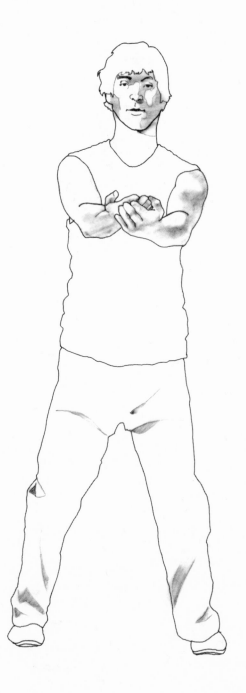

When you have reached
full upright position,
your hands and arms
should be extended
parallel to the ground.

Figure 86

Push your right hand
slightly out and pull
back your left hand
slightly.

Figure 87

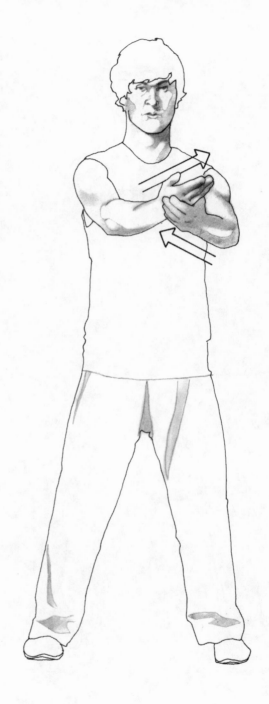

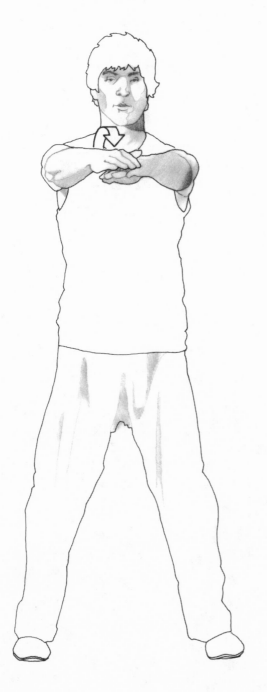

Turn your right hand over your left hand. Now both palms are turned downward.

Figure 88

Sit back and
slide your hands
slightly outward.
Return to the Map
of T'ai Chi.

Figure 89

Repeat the entire
form two more
times, from the
beginning.

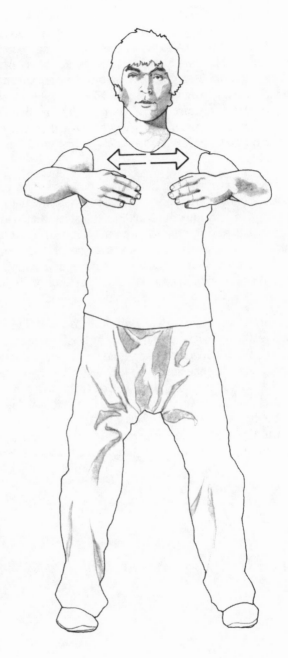

Spend at least one week on this form, particularly in conjunction with the preceding five forms. Time of execution for three repetitions should be two to five minutes. Doing it correctly is difficult. If you have trouble aligning your back, ask a friend to take a yardstick and hold it to your back from the coccyx up to the head. You want to try to align your spine like this when you reach the lowest point of the posture when your thighs are parallel to the ground. You can also practice looking backward into a mirror and slowly develop the sensitivity to know when your head and spine are aligned.

This exercise strengthens the bowels and genitals. It is of paramount importance to a healthy individual to keep their sexual energy in harmony with nature. Just as diet and exercise play an important role in physical and mental health, so too does the naturalness and sensitivity of sex energy. I use the term sex energy rather than sexuality because I am not addressing an issue of social and moral conduct, rather, I am speaking of the organs themselves and the effects on mind and body.

In this posture the kidneys and the adrenal glands, which are right above the kidneys, are also strongly stimulated. There is a strong relationship between these glands and the health of our sex organs. Since the old theories posit a transformation of sex energy to Chi, and a further transfer to a Chi body, there is a basic need to be sensitive to and correctly utilize our sexual forces. The how, when, and why is beyond the scope of this primer. However, the adrenalin in our bodies, its connection to sexual energy, and its potential for strength of mind, body, and spirit is indeed worthy of consideration.

Wind
The Gentle

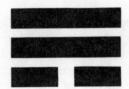

The
Rooting Exercise

"Meditation is the substance of wisdom;
wisdom is the function of meditation."
— Hui-neng

The rooting Exercise and Ascending Dragon are the last two of the basic forms. These can be learned and practiced together. Some Chinese boxing theoreticians insist that every stance is congruent to the horse. In fact, as I often did as a teacher of external arts, all stances are taught relative to the Horse. The Rooting Exercise is the full Horse stance as generally expounded in Chinese Martial Arts. It is congruent in form to the Short Horse stance learned while Holding the Ball. Ideally, the width of the stance is equal to twice the width of the shoulders. However, as in Holding the Ball, we keep the same inverted "U" shape, head and spine erect, weight at the bubbling well and knees not extending over the toes.

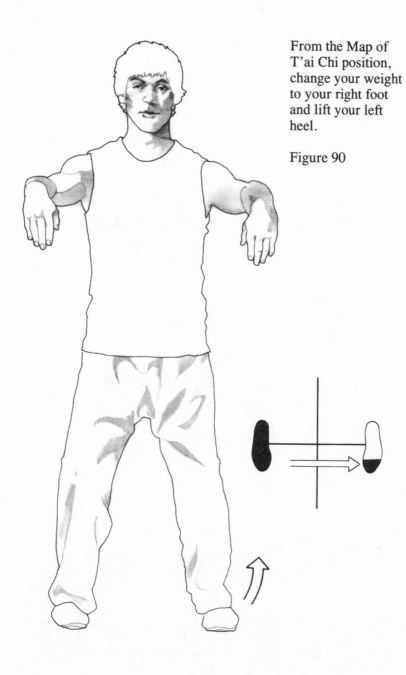

From the Map of
T'ai Chi position,
change your weight
to your right foot
and lift your left
heel.

Figure 90

Extend your arms outward, wrists relaxed. Look left, then step left with the toe touching first.

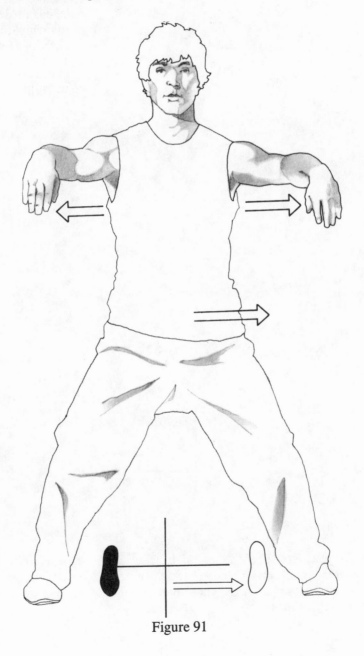

Figure 91

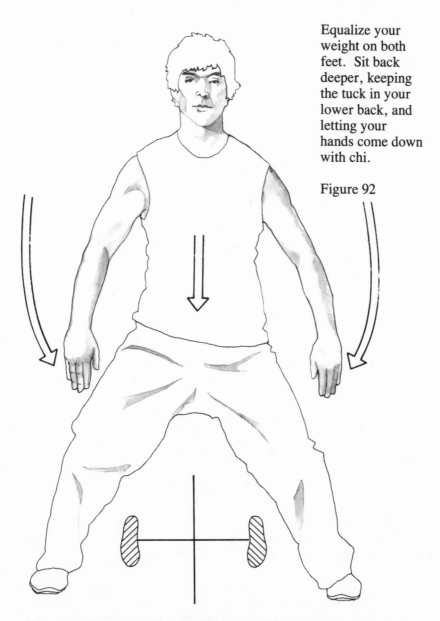

Equalize your weight on both feet. Sit back deeper, keeping the tuck in your lower back, and letting your hands come down with chi.

Figure 92

Now your feet should be parallel, about as far apart as twice your shoulder width and pointing straight ahead. You are seated as if you were riding a horse, knees bowed out slightly, but not extending over the toes.

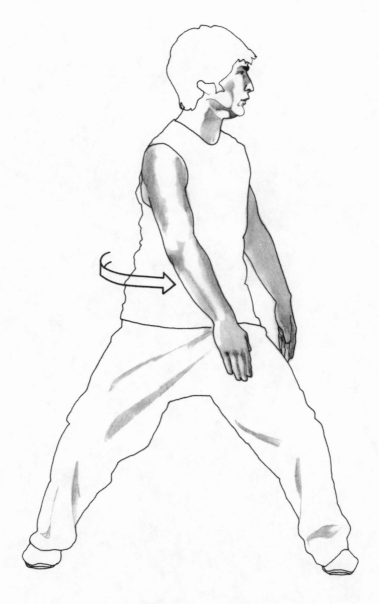

Figure 93

Keeping your back straight and not moving your knees, legs, or hips, rotate the waist 90° to your left. This movement is initiated and directed from the waist; do not turn only from your shoulders.

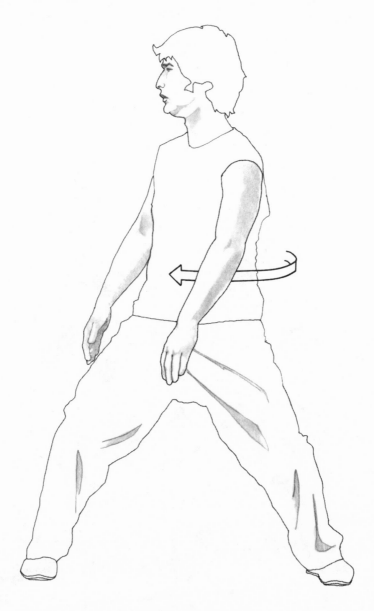

Figure 94

Now rotate from the waist 180° to your right.

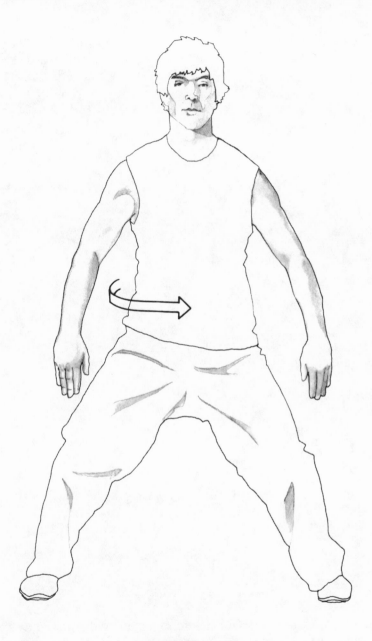

Figure 95

Rotate back 90° to the left, completing one full rotation.

Repeat the entire form at least twelve times, completing the turn to the right and left. You will finish facing forward.

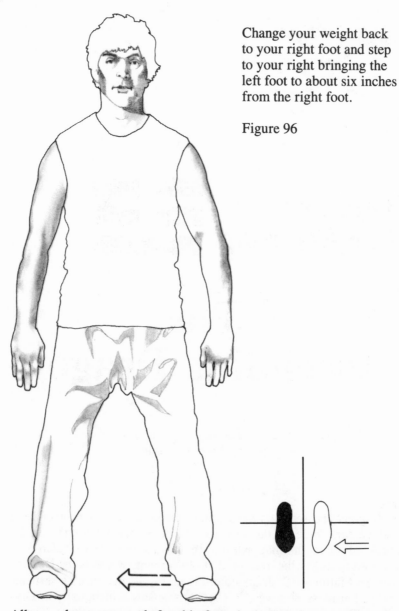

Change your weight back to your right foot and step to your right bringing the left foot to about six inches from the right foot.

Figure 96

Allow at least one week for this form including the preceding six. Twelve turns should take approximately two to six minutes. Remember not to put strength in your shoulders and to allow the waist to turn around your straight and supple spine. Sit low. Keep tucked and breathe abdominally. This posture aids in developing power in one's martial technique, yet at the same time massages and tonifies the inner organs below the diaphragm.

Thunder
The Arousing

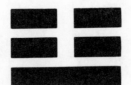

The
Ascending Dragon

"And as Moses lifted up the serpent into the wilderness,
even so must the Son of Man be lifted up."
— John 3:14

Dragons and serpents have often been associated with the Devil and the dark forces of the universe. Since no one has found one, we speak of them in imagination. In Revelations 10:16 Satan was referred to as "...the dragon, that old serpent, which is the Devil." Yet, in Matthew 10, Jesus counsels us to be "as wise as serpents and as harmless as doves." The Chinese saw a dichotomy in Dragons. Five-fingered dragons were considered benevolent. Three-fingered dragons were malevolent. I'm not certain that the number of fingers has much to do with good and bad; but I am certain that the sense of Jesus' words correlate to the Ascending Dragon form: have the wisdom to use all the principles fully and maintain a gentle softness. If you are stiff and rigid your three fingers may begin to show. Use your mind and body in a positive way; this is a further aspect of extending the Chi.

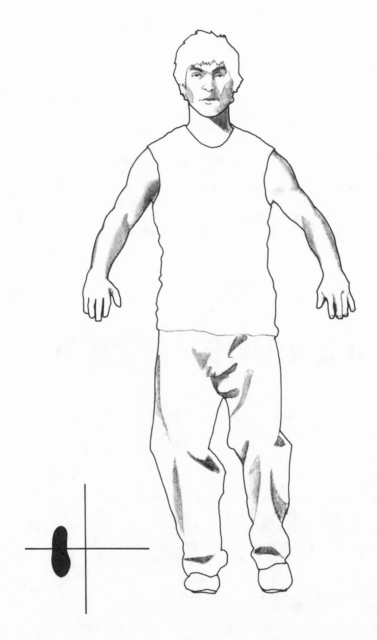

Figure 97

From the last position, sink a little on your right leg by bending the right knee.

Raise the whole body
up with the weight
on the right leg
while lifting up both
your left leg and
your arms. Continue
raising your arms and
left leg until your thigh
is parallel to the
ground and your left
foot points downward
next to your right leg.
Your hands should be
at eye level; your palms
facing down.

Figure 98

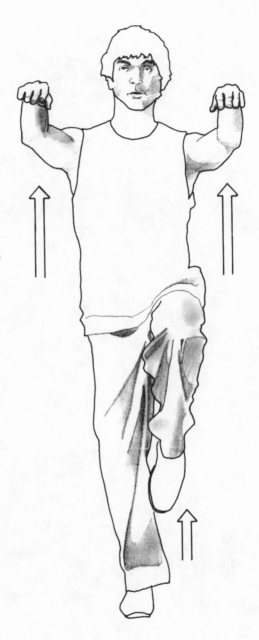

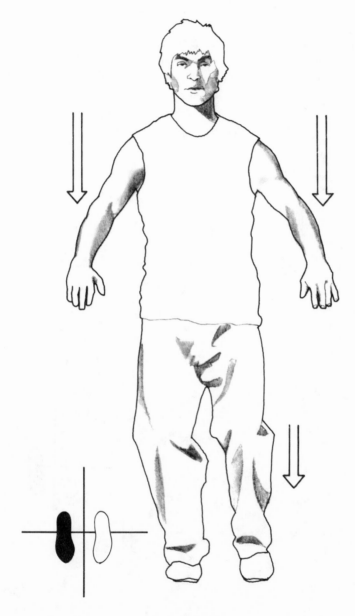

Figure 99

Gradually sink down on your right leg, lowering both your arms and left leg.

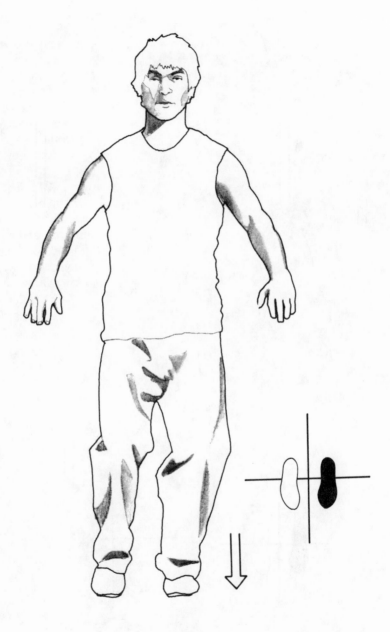

Figure 100

As your left toe touches the ground, gradually change weight to the left foot, keeping your left knee bent, sitting more on the left leg.

147

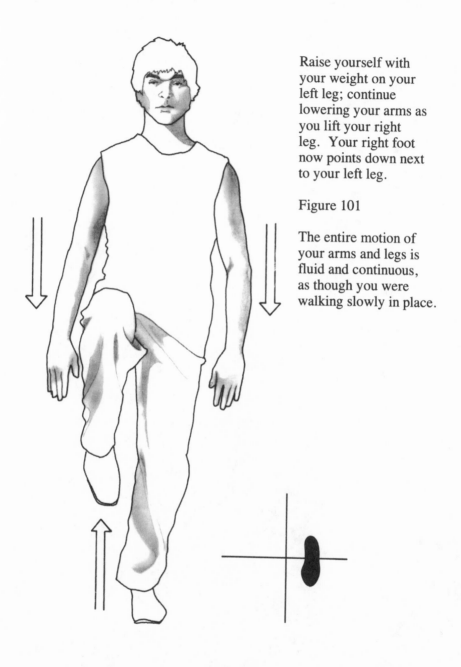

Raise yourself with your weight on your left leg; continue lowering your arms as you lift your right leg. Your right foot now points down next to your left leg.

Figure 101

The entire motion of your arms and legs is fluid and continuous, as though you were walking slowly in place.

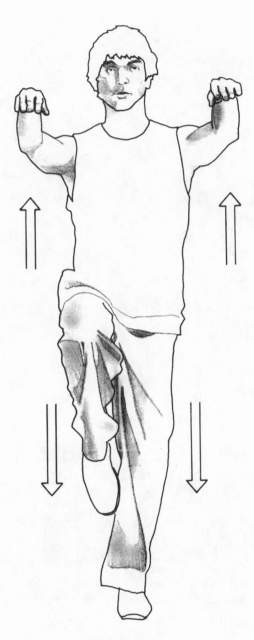

Figure 102

Sink down on your left leg as you bring your arms up and lower your right leg.

149

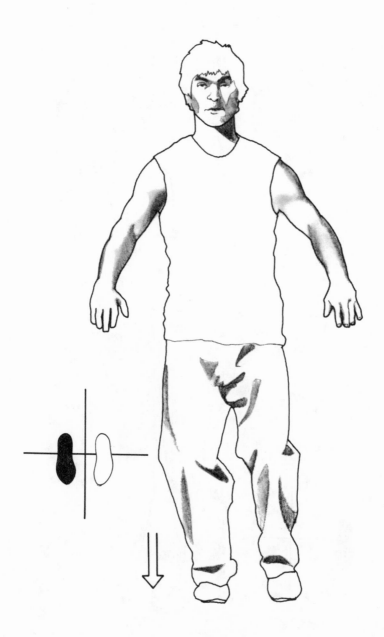

Figure 103

As your right toe touches down, gradually change your weight to the right foot and "sit" on the right leg.

Lift yourself up
with your weight
on your right leg,
bringing your left
leg and arms up.

Figure 104

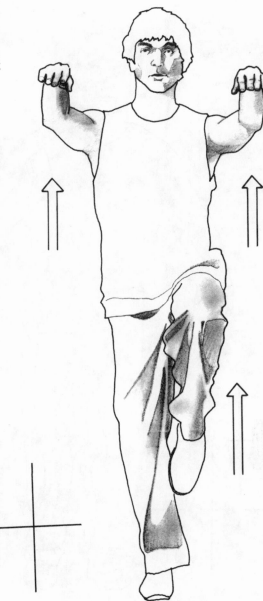

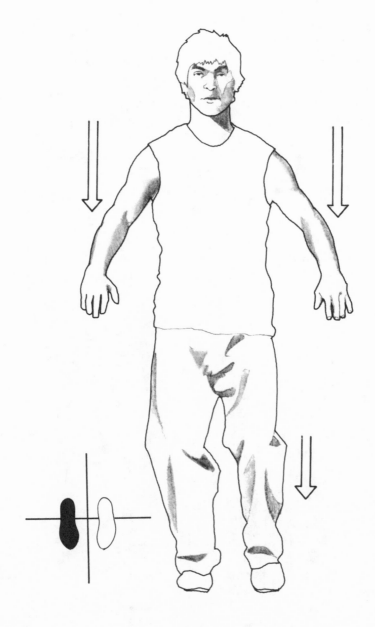

Figure 105

Sink again on the right leg as you lower your arms and left leg.

When your left toe touches down, change weight to the left foot.

Lift your body up on your left leg, bringing the right leg up and lowering your arms.

Figure 106

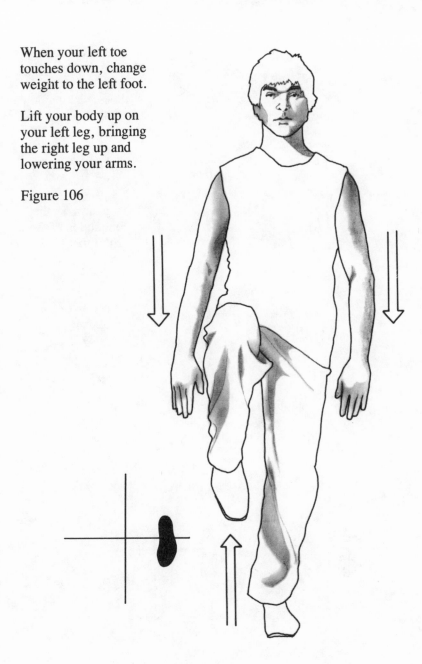

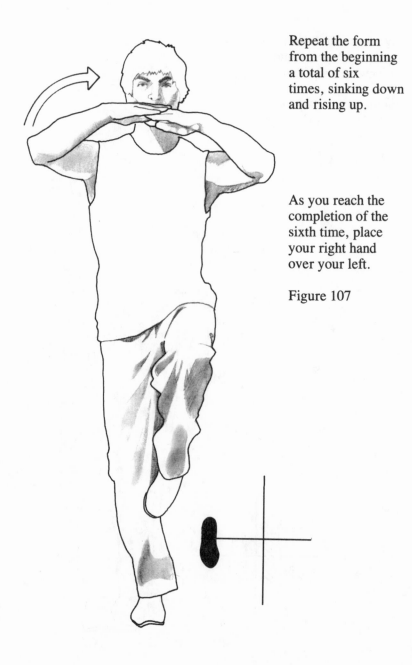

Repeat the form from the beginning a total of six times, sinking down and rising up.

As you reach the completion of the sixth time, place your right hand over your left.

Figure 107

As you bring the left leg
down, push your hands
downward and exhale.

Figure 108

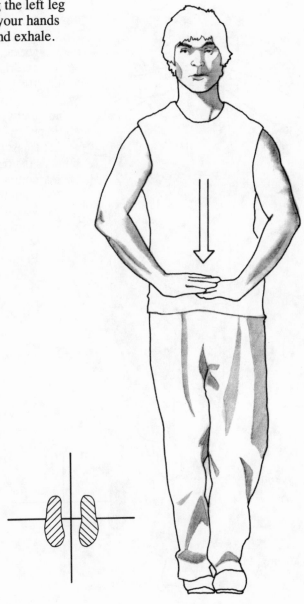

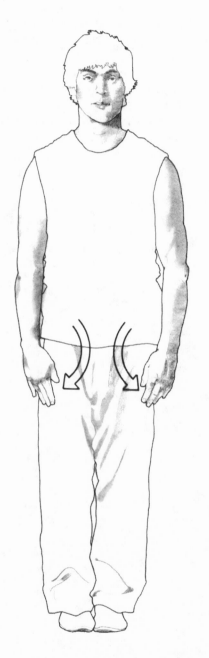

When your left toe touches down, your hands come to your sides as you equalize the weight on both feet.

Figure 109

Stand quietly and gather your energy for a minute or so. This last position is the same as the first position we learned.

The Ascending Dragon is the last of the Essential Movements. It is a good idea to allow another week for this form. As in all the forms, the movements are done in one smooth and continuous motion. This form with all repetitions may take two to four minutes. The whole set of movements including Preparation and Holding the Ball may take from fifteen to fifty minutes. Slowly, without straining, at about forty minutes is ideal. If you have only a few minutes, any of the eight forms may be done singularly, but always allow for the full number of repetitions.

Solo Exercises

All forms are imperfect, not in the sense that they are flawed, but rather that they have the ability to grow and improve. We must not discard the old solely for the sake of the new or retain the old and give no regard to what is new. In T'ai Chi all things are new and all things are old.

The Essential Movements we have studied are simple "solo" exercises; that is, a sequence of movements performed by an individual. A complete solo exercise is found in every school or style of T'ai Chi Ch'uan. Although these schools differ in expression and form, they all use the same principles and must have the same content to be called T'ai Chi. The core of principles is found in the *T'ai Chi Classics*.

All schools and styles of T'ai Chi use these Classics as a fundamental framework by which they develop content. The major schools of T'ai Chi Ch'uan are the Chen Family, the Yang School, the Wu School, the Wu and Hao, and the Sun School. Within each of these schools there may exist differences in frame or form, different styles, and shortened forms. For example, in the Yang School there are two separate forms. One is called the Family Form (T'ai Chi Chang Ch'uan), and the other is the T'ai Chi Ch'uan 108 as expounded by Yang Cheng Fu. From these forms there come various other shortened patterns. Observably, a T'ai Chi pattern or form consists of a series of movements. These individual movements may also be called forms.

The solo exercises of T'ai Chi Ch'uan are not only the basis for learning principles, but also an external manifestation of T'ai Chi. By developing within the context of the solo exercise, we improve not only ourselves, but all aspects of the Art. Furthermore, when seemingly unanswerable questions arise in the context of the art, or even in our daily lives, the solo exercise practice can be the key to unlock the riddles and paradoxes.

Though there are many styles and forms of T'ai Chi Ch'uan exercise, in principle they must all be the same to be considered true T'ai Chi Ch'uan. Far from being solely remnants of past wisdom, the Classics are indeed prophetic to each and every one who is a student of the Art. As one progresses, the Classics become the map of T'ai Chi and we can lean upon them to ask directions.

Besides the Classics, most of the Art has been handed down from generation to generation in an oral tradition. This accounts for the many styles and approaches, but we must keep in mind that the slightest deviation at the start of a long journey may lead us many miles from our destination, or completely off track. Even on the right track, it is possible to lose one's way; this accounts for the slowness in attaining T'ai Chi.

Fortunately, since the Path has become better travelled, we do have many good books that complement the Classics. Although the book, *Nine Secret Messages* by Ng Man Hap, published in November, 1967 in Hong Kong, is not by any means a "classic," Ng attributes the nine messages to Yang Lu Chan (1799-1872), whom many consider the foremost practitioner of modern day T'ai Chi. Yang Lu Chan gave the nine messages to his second son, Yang Pan Hou (1837-1892), who passed them down to Ng's teacher, Nin Lien Nien. Thanks to Mr. Hubert Lui for the translations from the Chinese texts.

On the Nine Secret Messages

The first message: *"The full application of T'ai Chi relies primarily on Chi; the body being relaxed, the Chi is gathered together, and the spirit is centered and high."*

Previously, we stated and hopefully have observed that T'ai Chi without Chi is not the true art. T'ai Chi demands not only faith in the Life Force, but also awareness, utilization, and application. Although modern science and philosophy have scoffed at the "miracles" of Christ as the "Christian Myth," these miracles are readily apparent and comprehensible in light of working with the Life Force, i.e., Chi. Of course, one needn't be religious or practice a particular martial art form to develop Chi. As long as the principles are maintained and developed, the Chi will be developed. The particular approach to this development as in a form of exercise is secondary, but nonetheless important. By concentrating or gathering together the Chi, we feel wonderful and hence our spirit is stable, centered, and high as in the sense of ecstasy.

The second message refers to the thirteen basic postures. These postures, or methods, reflect a simplicity of form from which we can develop a myriad of postures, forms, and movements, each and every one being a complete T'ai Chi. Furthermore, each and every T'ai Chi posture can be broken down into components of actions that directly correlate to the Thirteen Basic Postures or Methods. The Thirteen Basic Postures or Methods are given as follows:

Ward Off — P'eng. To Ward Off is to turn aside, avert, parry, or repel. "A trigger force of a mere four taels manages to move an object weighing one thousand catties."

Roll Back — Lu. To Roll Back is to reduce to a previous position, to retreat, to turn back. It is the employment of one side of the body with the purpose of directing and re-directing; it is yielding with purpose.

Press — Chi. To Press is to exert a heavy and steady force, to bear down on, or to squeeze. It is the use of rooting and Chin and not muscular force.

Push — An. To Push is to force away, to thrust or to urge forward. It is the use of rooting and Chin and not muscular force.

Pull — Ts'ai. To Pull is to remove from a fixed position, extract, or cause motion toward the source, to attract, to draw, or to withdraw. Often this action is called "Pull Down."

Split — Lieh. To separate, disunite, break, or divide sharply constitutes the action of Split. To Split does not mean to divide or disunite your own action, but to do the various postures that would have a dividing effect on an adversary.

Elbow — Tsou. Using the elbow requires the notion of Folding. To Fold Up is to make compact by bending at the joint, to bring from an extended to a closed position, to place together or to envelop. The basic posture is Strike with Elbow, but Folding can be done at any of the joints.

Shoulder — K'ao. Using the shoulder requires the notion of Release. To Release is to let go, to set free from restraint, to relinquish or to unfasten. The basic posture is called Release Shoulder, or Shoulder Stroke, but it is the action of releasing and non-attachment that is fundamental.

Advance. To move forward or to a forward position, or to move onward, describes the action of Advance. We should note that it is possible to step backward and still advance, as in the case of moving backward while our focus is forward, or our Chi extends forward. The T'ai Chi Classics emphasize the idea that in advance there must also be a retreat and in retreat, there must also be an advance.

Retreat. The act of going backward or withdrawing describes the action of Retreat. In T'ai Chi the action of Retreat does not imply submission, but rather an action of mobility that puts one in a desirable position.

Shift to Right; Shift to Left. Looking Right or Left relies on Yielding and the ability to neutralize. To give way to force or pressure, to empty one side of the body, is the T'ai Chi action of Yielding. This does not mean to be overcome or be defeated. In the Thirteen Basic Postures, Yielding is considered in two directions, Look to Right and Gaze to Left. However, we are concerned with the action itself, hence this notion of Yielding includes both these directions as singular aspects. Unlike the action of Roll Back or Pull, there is no implication of re-direction. It is purely Yielding. Unlike Retreat, there need not be backward movement. This is lateral movement to complement advance and retreat.

Central Equilibrium. The action of Centering, taking root, in one's posture, stability, or the canceling of all acting forces around that center denotes the action of Central Equilibrium. All other actions must be performed through the action of Central Equilibrium, or you will not have control of their entire functions. This final posture, therefore, includes the ability to neutralize and make the adverse force ineffective.

Although the simplicity of older T'ai Chi forms that relied heavily on the expressions of these basic postures is gone, we may at least look at the second message: *"In the Thirteen Basic Postures, the ability to change is the key."* This means change and transformation of one into the other. One must understand how Ward Off becomes Roll Back, or how Retreat becomes Advance. Hence, the transformations are as equally important as the postures themselves. One cannot observe principles only at the start and culmination of a posture, but indeed at every point in between. Transformation is change.

The third message tells us: *"In Yee (will), the mind is essential. To improve the Art in variation and change is to widen the scope in ways of application. T'ai Chi has no fixed Way. The Way is moving and changing."*

The distinction between the Mind and the Will is well taken. But in T'ai Chi one's Will and one's Mind work in harmony. Modern English allows for the equivocal use of the words "brain" and "mind." The brain is a physical organ that governs our physical body in the sense of control and direction, and creating the electro-chemical impulses that travel through the entire body via the nervous system. Modern science often views the Mind as a function of the Brain. This certainly is a truth, but not a complete truth since the brain is also a function of the mind.

The author recognizes the seeming paradoxes that Mind and Body are one and yet we must speak often in terms of Mind and Body as being different. The oneness of Mind and Body is harmonious oneness, as in the sense of Yin and Yang. The differentiation of Mind and Body is apparent through our experiences. Through our mind we may understand variation and change, thereby seeing many types of applications regarding various postures and the Art as a whole. Thus, due to the principle of change, we may say that T'ai Chi has no rigid, singular approach and where there is an approach, it is as Heraclitus would say, "in the state of flux."

The fourth message: *"Firmness and emptiness: where ever there is hardness within softness, your situation is impregnable."*

Hard and soft are, of course, Yin and Yang. Only by achieving the harmony of the complementary opposites, hard and soft, do we have T'ai Chi. If an outside Yang tries to disturb our harmony, it will be taken up by our Yin. If an outside Yin appears on the horizon, it receives our Yang. Thus, being able to meet and respond to any stimulus and at the same time retain our harmonious oneness, one's situation is locked-up and impregnable. This is readily apparent in T'ai Chi's martial applications, the outside Yang may be a punch or kick at our mid-section, to which our soft, yielding quality neutralizes and therefore controls. An outside Yin may be a retreat to which our Yang extension of Chi, as in the case of a push, repels and thwarts the opponent.

The fifth message: *"Mixed circles: to retreat or yield, be empty. To advance or extend, be solid. Then your strength is based on the art of your spiral movement."*

163

It is interesting to note that in the circle we may see the Infinite. Yet a circle also consists of Yin and Yang, outside and inside, right side and left side, upper and lower, the latter two being the semicircular components of a circle. Therefore, the circular, arc-like or spiraling movements that characterize T'ai Chi also express the theory of Yin and Yang.

The sixth message further responds: *"The art of confused circles is most difficult to comprehend. However, its changes and variations are mysteriously unlimited."*

The term "confused circles" does not mean that you must be confused about how your hands and movements circle. It is termed confused because an observer watching the mixed circularity cannot comprehend their beginning or ends or directions. The practitioner, however, must be fully aware of the implications and applications of each and every circular movement.

The seventh message warns us: *"Very few people are devoted to the study of Yin and Yang in T'ai Chi. Its technique lies in the knowledge of contracting and expanding, opening and closing, hard and soft, side and corner, activity and inactivity, increase and decrease, retreat and advance, light and firm, solid and empty . . ."*

The eighth message refers to the Eighteen Basics, including the Thirteen Basic Postures, and also says: *"Calm [wait for the opportunity], Not Impeded [due to double-weightedness], Smooth [unified and light], Empty [to guard], Solid [to charge]."*

These last five ideas refer to attitude. A martial artist, for example, will never go beyond the level of a novice unless he learns to wait, not be double-weighted, be soft and confident, not pay any mind to the stimulus, and thereby be able to respond naturally to any attack, and finally, immediately integrate one's entire being in the counter-attack.

The ninth message intones: *"Roundness of movement is essential."*

Like softness, roundness has no opposite in T'ai Chi except for its natural complementary opposite. There must not be any sharp angles or linear projections. In softness, there is no hard, tense movement of the body that would violate the principle of relaxation, yet in terms of its complementary opposite, hardness means extension of one's Chi. Likewise, in roundness, there can be no sharp angles or linear projections, but the complementary opposite of linearity is often termed the curve seeking to be straight.

Commentary on the Nine Secret Messages

The idea of secrecy has long been embedded in the cultural heritage of T'ai Chi Ch'uan. The Chen clan taught no one outside their village for generations. Many T'ai Chi teachers with advanced and sophisticated methods of training took their "secrets" to their graves. But the biggest secret of all is that there is no secret and this is no secret at all.

Heaven cannot be seen because it is so vast. Where, then, is the need for secrets? As a personal note, I caution every aspiring student of T'ai Chi to beware of secrets, secret styles, and secret Masters. Nothing is better than correct principle. T'ai Chi is the Teacher of us all, and T'ai Chi loves every student equally. Natural talent is not a guarantee of success; perseverance and proper instruction are.

The Three Inner Schools

In the Nine Messages attributed to Yang Lu Chan we are not surprised to see the emphasis on circularity. Pa Kua Chang, Eight Trigram Palm (the sister art of T'ai Chi Ch'uan along with Hsing-I Ch'uan, Mind-Form Boxing), is the greatest exponent of circularity. Since the principles governing T'ai Chi, Pa Kua and Hsing-I are identical, it seems that learning any one of them would be sufficient as a lifelong end. This is true, but it is also true that they can be seen as three links of a circular chain that comprise the inner schools of Chinese pugilism, yoga, and meditation.

What T'ai Chi students can beneficially derive from Pa Kua is indeed the emphasis on circularity. The entire form is done in a circle, much like a European or American Indian folk dance. Every hand movement is circular, arc-like, and spiraling. There are several things that studying Pa Kua does to aid students of T'ai Chi Ch'uan. First it teaches, in depth, the art of stepping and walking. In practice it is often performed as though one is trodding through deep mud, careful in stepping as not to splatter or make undue noise.

Second, it emphasizes circular and spiral rotation, in and from the waist. This greatly loosens and stretches the muscles around the waist, and further tonifies the internal organs. Third, the martial enthusiasts learn the formal applications of the palm. And fourth, the student is forced to make measurements in completely circular terms. The size of the step and the diameter of the circle change the positions of the forms.

Pa-Kua is based on the theory of the Eight Trigrams, which are devised by taking the two components of T'ai Chi, Yin and Yang, in combinations of three at a time, yielding the eight trigrams. The Eight Trigrams taken in combinations of two at a time yield the sixty-four hexagrams that compose the notion of change in Chinese philosophical thought. Hsing-I-Ch'uan is based on the theory of the five elements. The ancient Chinese did not consider the universe to be composed of only five elements, rather they thought that all of the elements found in our plane of existence could fall into five basic categories: earth, wood, metal, fire, water. In Hsing-I the T'ai Chi student may learn, in greater depth, the importance of not only learning how to move, but also of how to be still and thereby realize that mind contains and creates form.

Martial Art Application

If we were to characterize each specific posture as having a particular martial art application, we would be limited. In T'ai Chi, strikes may often be interpreted as parries; there are no "blocks" in T'ai Chi Ch'uan. Postures or defensive movements can be equally interpreted as offensive movements. Indeed, true martial art is situational and it is the artist that must rise to the situation. For example, if someone were to punch towards the side of my head, I would not ask them to wait a moment so I could correctly position my body and respond to their attack with a classical defensive counter. The response to any attack must be immediate, without forethought and be the correct response to that particular situation. Thereby, the old Chinese saying, "the Master may be struck down by the blind fist," has a profound meaning.

The martial art techniques found in the solo exercise have a multitude of variations, a different variation to correspond to each and every martial situation. Therefore, understanding applications is important for each and every T'ai Chi form. Since each T'ai Chi form has many different applications, we must be primarily concerned with the internal situation and not the external form.

Much of T'ai Chi Ch'uan is learned on a subconscious level. Attaining just a small degree of mastery means that the walls between the conscious and subconscious minds have been broken down. This is also the elimination of doubt. Breaking down the walls between conscious and subconscious thought is a vital part of good mental health, as well as T'ai Chi Ch'uan.

In doing the solo exercise, if we envision it as purely a martial art form and see myriads of opponents before us, we will have violated the principle of relaxation and harmony. It is also incorrect to lose sight of the martial values, for in doing so, we are exposed and self-ishly depend on others to protect us.

Yet, the pinnacle of T'ai Chi Ch'uan involves neither offense nor defense. It is like Daniel walking into the lion's den without a weapon, calmly and confidently. The raging lions also become calm and loving. Furthermore, martial arts is not to defend oneself only against a physical aggressor, but more readily to protect ourselves from physical, mental, or spiritual disease.

Physicians in China have often used singular T'ai Chi postures coordinated with breathing to cure a multitude of maladies. The singular postures were repeated over and over again at different times of the day, and were designed to specifically affect the area in question. The focus was not on curing the symptom, but rather on allowing the body to heal itself and eventually eliminate the cause. It is interesting to note that movements done singularly are an integral part of the T'ai Chi boxers' method of training: one movement done many times with coordinated breathing, one movement done many times continuously. The minimum number of times was usually ten. Once again we note the parallels between health and martial art.

The revived interest in Classical Chinese medicine has established countless approaches to the ideas of acupuncture, herbology, acupressure and so on. But these arts of medicine have an incomplete worth without the notion of Chi. A good physician must also develop his own Chi, thereby enabling him to either heal others or help them heal themselves. Whether a doctor is of the Eastern or Western persuasion, the intensity of his or her Chi is directly correlated to the ability to heal.

It shouldn't surprise us that much of T'ai Chi principle is based on Classical Chinese philosophy. At the top of the list would be the *Tao Teh Ching* and the *I Ching* which form the cornerstones for Classical philosophy of ancient China. The parallels of these philosophical texts are understandably seen in Christianity, Buddhism, Judaism, Islam, etc. There are also principle analogies to Socratic, Platonic, and even Aristotelean thought. T'ai Chi is not a religion, yet it encompasses the philosophical truths of all religions, or better yet, their principles.

At the core of T'ai Chi is the philosophy of Yin and Yang. Yin and Yang are the complementary opposites of T'ai Chi, yet within Yin there is Yang and within Yang there is Yin. Furthermore, within the Yin that lies in the Yang, there is another Yang and within that Yang, another Yin and so forth, ad infinitum.

The key is change, but not change in the normal connotation of the word. Here change is not mere change. Often we hear the adage, "all things change." But if all things change, then that very fact must, by definition, change. This is a ridiculous contradiction. The change of T'ai Chi is the Universal Flow, in the sense of Heraclitus who said, "All things (the universe) flow."

I respectfully ask you to consider why one should study T'ai Chi. If it is for health, meditation, martial arts, philosophy, or beautiful movement, I can understand this. Again I must ask, my friends, why one should study T'ai Chi? An old story has it that the disciple of a master decided to explore new heights. He left his old master and went up into the mountains to study with the immortals for twenty years. One day he decided to pay a visit to his old master and sought him out in his former home. They met each other with open arms and decided to revisit their old place of meditation. The new master told his old teacher that in the mountains he had aspired to heaven. As they came to a river on their short journey, the old man got onto the ferry and gave the boatman his fare. The younger master was dismayed and showing his great skill, simply walked across the water. Upon reaching the shore he asked his old teacher, "Master, why did you take the ferry and not just walk across the water?" The old master looked at him happily and replied, "Did you study for twenty years just to save a nickel?"

It has been over ten years since I began to jot down notes that have taken the form of this text. I recognize it to be with God's help since my understanding is limited. I encourage future generations to expand to new horizons, I believe we can unravel the mysteries enjoyably. I caution my friends to not confuse the finger with the moon nor mistake the plate for the meal.

Tsao Li Ming likened the study of T'ai Chi to walking along a beautiful path that had no beginning and no end. Enjoy the walk.